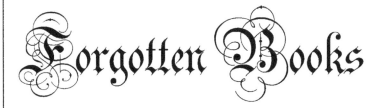

ISBN 978-0-243-06204-1
PIBN 10785593

FB &c Ltd, Dalton House, 60 Windsor Avenue, London, SW19 2RR.
Company number 08720141. Registered in England and Wales.

For support please visit www.forgottenbooks.com

1 MONTH OF
FREE
READING

at
www.ForgottenBooks.com

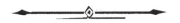

By purchasing this book you are eligible for one month membership to ForgottenBooks.com, giving you unlimited access to our entire collection of over 1,000,000 titles via our web site and mobile apps.

To claim your free month visit:

www.forgottenbooks.com/free785593

F DIABETESMELL
SENAUR
ITSELF TO BE A
VE SPECIF

UST BE USED PROPERL

half tumbler of water (three times daily, after
y 6 drops), and increasing one drop each day.
iined by pushing Arsenauro and Mercauro to po
se (keeping the patient as near that point as possi
ridely, some patients taking eighty-five drops three
ach a dose of over ten drops.
eration, (manifested by the usual signs, such as pu
vacuations, frontal headache, dizziness, tingling
ld be stopped for twenty-four hours, then resume
dministered when toleration point was reached. I
ascertained limit for a protracted period.

A "Flannel Blanket" Tongue.

"Milk is all right at times," said Dr. B—, "but take a case with a tongue like a fuzzy flannel blanket and milk will but add to the trouble."

Liquid Peptonoids is a valuable nutrient when milk cannot be given. It is pre-digested—absorbable—aseptic.

One to two tablespoonfuls.

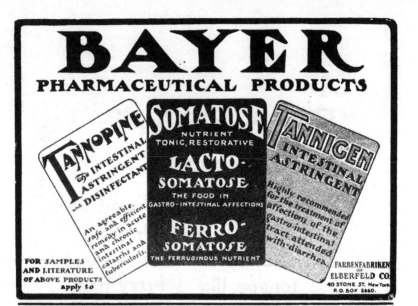
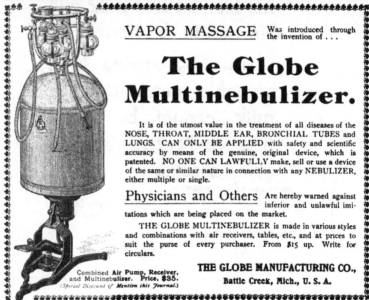

Professional Directory.

HOURS: 11-12, 3-5. TELEPHONE 1366.

H. C. CROWELL, M. D.

Gynaecology and Abdominal Surgery.

Altman Bldg., 11th and Walnut Sts.,

KANSAS CITY, MO.

John H. Thompson, M. D.

Ophthalmic Surgeon,

DEARDORFF BLDG.,

KANSAS CITY, MO.

Office Hours: TELEPHONE 2286.

8:00 a. m. to 12:30 p. m.
2:00 p. m. to 4:00 p. m.

DR. HAL FOSTER

Practice Limited to Throat, Nose and Ear.

Rooms 402, 403 and 404 ALTMAN BLDG.,

S. E. Cor. 11th and Walnut Sts.,

KANSAS CITY, MO

TELEPHONE { OFFICE 618.
RES. SOUTH 144.

Herman E. Pearse, M. D.

SURGEON,

322-323 Rialto Bldg.

OFFICE HOURS: 2 TO 5 P. M. KANSAS CITY, MO.

JOHN W. PERKINS, M. D.

SURGEON.

Office, Nos. 409, 410, 411 Altman Bldg.,

KANSAS CITY, MO.

Office: Altman Bldg., 11th and Walnut. Residence: 2901 Forest Avenue

JOHN PUNTON, M. D.

PRACTICE LIMITED TO

Nervous and Mental Diseases.

KANSAS CITY, MO.

A. H. Cordier, M. D.

Prof. Abdominal Surgery in University Medical College.

Practice Limited to

Diseases of Women and Abdominal Surgery.

Office, Rialto Bldg., Kansas City, Mo.

Dr. John M. Langsdale

LIMITS HIS PRACTICE TO

Genito-Urinary, Venereal and Skin Diseases.

OFFICE, 509-10 ALTMAN BUILDING

S. E. COR. 11th AND WALNUT STS

Professional Directory.

DR. MILO B. WARD.

SURGERY AND DISEASES OF WOMEN.

OFFICE:

RIALTO BLDG., KANSAS CITY, MO.

Dr. Emory Lanphear,

Practice Limited to

Surgery and Gynaecology,

4049 FINNEY AVE.,

ST. LOUIS, MO.

DR. WM. FRICK,

LECTURER DERMATOLOGY,
KANSAS CITY MEDICAL COLLEGE.

OFFICE ROOM, 301 RIALTO BUILDING.

OFFICE HOURS:,
10 to 12 A. M.,
4 to 5 P. M.

Special attention given
to Skin and Venereal
Diseases.

HOURS { 9 to 12 a. m.
2 to 4 p. m. TEL. { Res., West 176
Office 1249

Dr. J. E. Sawtell,

NOSE, THROAT
AND CHEST.......

Rooms 310-311 Rialto Building

Kansas City, Mo.

S. GROVER BURNETT, M. D.

Electro Therapy, Mental and Nervous Diseases.

425 Rialto,

9-12 and 3 5.
Telephone 1017. Kansas City, Mo.

Office Hours,
9—12
1— 4

TEL. 1991.

W. H. Schutz, M. D.

EYE AND EAR SURGEON

Rooms 307-308 Rialto Building,

KANSAS CITY, MO.

TELEPHONE,

OFFICE HOURS:
10 to 12 A. M.
1 to 4.30 P. M.

F. H. Clark, M. D.

SPECIAL ATTENTION GIVEN
TO MEDICAL ELECTRICITY.

539--540 NEW RIDGE BUILDING
KANSAS CITY, MO.

OFFICE HOURS:
9:00 to 12:00 A. M.
4:00 to 5:00 P. M.

Telephone 744.

Jabez N. Jackson, M. D.

SURGEON.

Office 529-30 Rialto Building, 9th and Grand
Avenue.

WALNUT LODGE,

A Private Hospital for the Special Treatment of ALCOHOL and
OPIUM INEBRIATES.

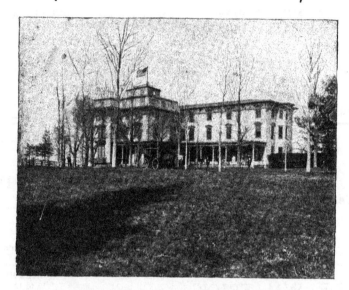

THIS Institution was founded in 1878 on the modern view that INEBRIETY is a DISEASE and CURABLE. Each patient is made the subject of special study, and SPECIAL MEDICAL TREATMENT SUITED TO THE EXACT REQUIREMENTS OF THE CASE. The general plan of treatment is building up the diseased organism and restoring both mind and body to a healthy and normal condition, with BRAIN and NERVE, REST, ETC. This is accomplished by TURKISH, RUSSIAN, and SALINE BATHS, ELECTRICITY, MASSAGE, tonics, diet, and every other means known to science and experience which have proven to be of value in these cases.

This Hospital is pleasantly situated in the suburbs with the best surroundings and every appointment of an elegant residence

Experience proves that a large proportion of cases who come under treatment, and who unite with the physician in the use of all means of treament, are permanently restored and cured. Each case has the direct personal care of the physician and attendant; and no one is received for less than four months unless by special arrangement.

All letters and inquiries should be addressed,

T. D. CROTHERS, M.D., Hartford, Conn.

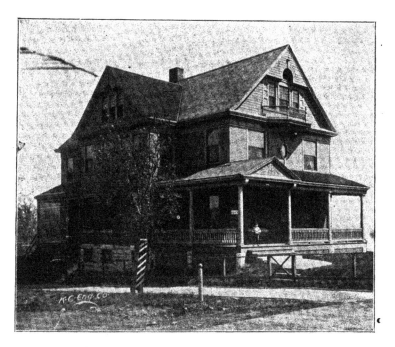

A Private Home

for Nervous Invalids.

A limited number of patients will be received at my residence for the care and treatment of Nervous and Mental Diseases requiring *Isolation*. Elegant location combined with all the latest modern conveniences. One block from Troost Park—Inspection desired

References:—The Medical Profession of Kansas City and Vicinity.

Address

JOHN PUNTON, M. D.

KANSAS CITY, MO.

OFFICE:	RESIDENCE:
Altman Building,	**2901 Forest Avenue,**
11th and Walnut St	**Telephone 337.**

Please mention the Journal when you write to an advertiser.

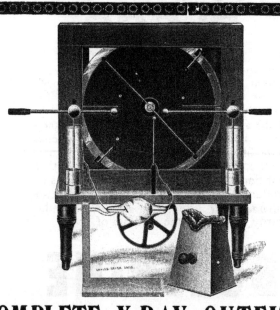

S. GROVER BURNETT, A. M., M. D.,

RECEIVES IN PRIVACY A LIMITED NUMBER OF CASES

OF THE

Drug Habit, Nervous Diseases and Mild Mental Diseases.

OPIUM, CHLORAL AND COCAINE CASES ARE
ESPECIALLY DESIRED.

REFERENCE BY PERMISSION:

LANDON CARTER GRAY, M. D., Prof. Mental and Nervous Diseases, N. Y. Polyclinic.
GRAEME M. HAMMOND, M. D., Prof. Mental and Nervous Diseases, New York Post-Graduate Medical College.
WILLIAM J. MORTON, M. D., Prof. Electro Therapeutics and Mental and Nervous Diseases, New York Post-Graduate Medical College.
FREDERICK PETERSON, M. D., Chief Vanderbilt Clinic, Neurological Dept., College Physicians and Surgeons, New York City.
WILLIAM L. LESZYNSKY, M. D., Neurologist to Demilt Dispensary, New York City.

Address, Rialto Building, 9th St. and Grand Ave., Kansas City, Mo.

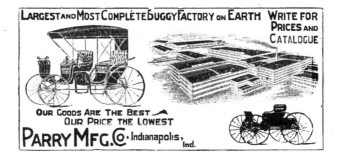

ANTIKAMNIA & QUININE LAXATIVE TABLETS
IN COLDS - FEVER - MALARIA
FIVE-GRAIN ANTIKAMNIA TABLETS
IN ALL NERVE & MUSCLE-PAIN
ANTIKAMNIA & CODEINE TABLETS
IN COUGHS-ACUTE & CHRONIC
ANTIKAMNIA & QUININE TABLETS
IN CORYZA - LA GRIPPE - ETC
MADE SOLELY BY
THE ANTIKAMNIA
CHEMICAL COMPANY
ST. LOUIS, U.S.A.
SEND US YOUR CARD AND WATCH RESULTS

Satyria

SATYRIA

TRADE MARK—REGISTERED.

THE IDEAL

GENITO-URINARY TONIC AND NERVE RECONSTITUENT.

It Fulfills All the Demands which Can be Made Upon It.

Sample and Literature Furnished upon Request Accompanied by Professional Card and on Payment of Express Charges.

FORMULA:

Saw Palmetto, False Bitter Sweet, Couch Grass, Moyra Pauma, Phosphorus, Syrup and Aromatics.

SATYRIA PHARMACAL CO.,

ST. LOUIS, MO., U. S. A.

W. A. Charman, Sole Proprietor.

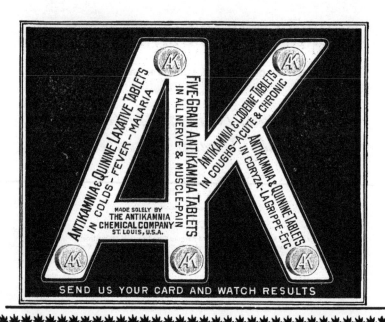

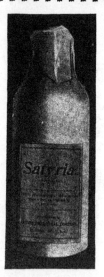

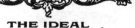

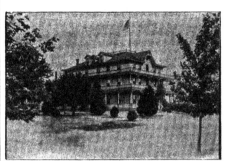
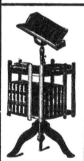
—13—

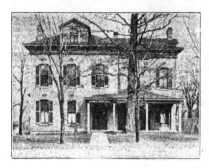
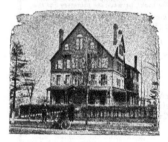
—14—

NERVOUS INSTABILITY,

impaired co-ordination, insomnia, disordered digestion, and the protean neurotic manifestations which make up the symptom-group of Neurasthenia are all, according to a recent writer, "**primarily anæmic**" in origin. It logically follows, therefore, that the essential therapeutic indication is to "build up" and enrich the blood——

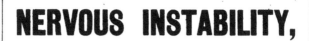

IRON AND MANGANESE
IN NEUTRAL ORGANIC COMBINATION

provides a readily available pabulum for corpuscular nutrition, and increase and by supplying vital force to the blood stream also feeds and vivifies the nervous system, establishes physiological equilibrium and restores nervous equipoise.

To assure the proper filling of prescriptions,
order Pepto-Mangan "Gude" in original bottles (℥ xi).
NEVER SOLD IN BULK.

M. J. BREITENBACH COMPANY,

Agents for American Continent,

LABORATORY,   (Tarrant Building), 100 WARREN STREET,
LEIPZIG, GERMANY.   **NEW YORK.**

THE KANSAS CITY
MEDICAL INDEX-LANCET.

A MONTHLY MAGAZINE OF MEDICINE AND SURGERY.

——BY——

JOHN PUNTON, M. D., EDITOR AND PUBLISHER.

PUBLICATION OFFICE, 532 ALTMAN BUILDING, KANSAS CITY, MISSOURI.

All communications to THE INDEX-LANCET must be contributed to it exclusively. The Editor is not responsible for the views of contributors. Each contributor of an original article is entitled to a reasonable number of extra copies of THE INDEX-LANCET. Reprints of papers will be furnished at cost, orders for which must accompany manuscript. All communications should be addressed to the Editor.

ENTERED AT THE POSTOFFICE IN KANSAS CITY, MISSOURI, AS SECOND CLASS MAIL MATTER.

VOL. XXI. No. 5. MAY, 1900. WHOLE NUMBER 245

ORIGINAL CONTRIBUTIONS.

*ANNUAL ADDRESS.

BY H. C. CROWELL. M. D.

Professor of Gynecology University Medical College, Kansas City, Mo.

Mr. President and fellows of the Western Surgical and Gynecological Association, I should be unmindful indeed, if, at this time, I did not express to you my sincere thanks for the honor which I have enjoyed, of being your President, for the year 1899. I say this not in a perfunctory sense, but with genuine heart-felt sincerity; for the time has arrived, when, to be President of this Association, is to be President of one of the most influential Associations of this country, and permit me to digress, just enough, at this moment, to say that the time has past, when we must look to the East, only, for all that is good, either in business or professional attainments. The West is to-day setting the pace in all things, and may the Western Surgical and Gynecological Association be at the front.

Some Things.

Conforming to establish custom, I am expected as your President to deliver an address upon this occasion. I shall disappoint, or gratify, you by departing in some essentials from usual style and character of address, and content myself by briefly referring to some things which might, in my opinion, profitably occupy the thought of the Medical Profession. I shall not attempt more than to bring the questions before you, leaving the discussions largely for others who may be so disposed. There are many things practical to us as a profession, people and nation, that might be considered with profit to us collectively, but, since it cannot benefit any single individual by agitating these questions, it is safe to say they will remain but imperfectly considered.

At the recent Hereford Cattle Show, held in Kansas City with its large number of fine cattle, excellent and perfected in every particular, over the ordinary every day common breed, I was forcibly impressed with the degree of excellence, to which these cattle had been brought, but the attainment of

* Annual address delivered by the President of the Western Surgical and Gynecological Association at Des Moines, Iowa, December 28, 1899.

this degree of perfection, did not so occupy my mind, as the means employed to bring about such ends. And I could not refrain from making comparison, with the development of a people, the intelligence, the power, the agency of greatest import in carrying out the destiny of creation. How neglected, how utterly disregarded, are all laws for higher and more perfect development, when applied to the human race. Is it less important that the most potent factor in making history, man, should receive less thought and care in his pedigree than the dumb beasts, his slaves? Such we are compelled to admit is the case. In the case of the animal we look carefully to his pedigree, we know to an absolute certainty, what degree of purity his or her blood contains. Perfection is sought in every particular. The conture, temperament, durability, nature and peculiar class attributes are sought out in both, the male and female, in order that their union may produce the most typical specimen of their kind. The care given the progeny of well selected antecedents, is directed to the end of perfecting and developing to their fullest capabilities, their inherent possibilities; no detail is neglected; in seeking to perpetuate their kind, only the most perfect, according to a critical examination, are set apart for this purpose.

If this higher degree of development and perfection is desirable in the dumb beasts, in creatures that figure but in a material way, in the perpetuating of worlds, how much more should it seem, that some regard should be paid to the rules governing development and perpetuation by the human race? Why such utter disregard of all laws of development and improvement among men? We should remember, that the progeny, always corresponds to its progenitors; that its tendency is to degenerate rather than to improve, generation after generation, unless care is exercised to introduce improved blood on one side or the other. If the blood of one parent is tainted with some infirmity, weakness or pecularity, it is quite apt to be visited upon their progeny. In the human family, we observe none of the precautions taken by the cattle breeder, here chaos reigns supreme. No laws, no rules, no custom or thought governs in the selection of mates in the human family. The only governing factors are passion, fancy and fortune, either of which, outweigh any physical or mental consideration. The phthisical are joined to the phthisical, the neurotic to the neurotic, the viscious to the viscious, and so on through the category of inheritable features, until we have become a nation of cripples, dyspeptics and neurotics, inferior in stature and durability, if not intellectually. Such being the case, then, to a greater or less degree, should we not learn a lesson, from the grower of the lower animals, and insist that such rules and regulations be established as shall aid, at least, in stamping out inherited vices and disease, and bring about a higher order of beings; beings with better mental and physical constitutions. This is a political question which will, perforce, interest those who come after us, if it does not us; for the tendency is, by the permiscuous marrying and inter-marrying, regardless, to a degeneracy of the race, which in time, must effect a nation. Indeed, it may be truthfully said that to this cause, more than any other, may be attributed the fact that the descendants of Julius Caesar have degenerated to the banana seller, those of Demosthenes to the candy venders of our streets and the descendants of the mighty Moore relegated to the deserts of Africa. Let us have laws which shall prevent flagrant violations of all physiological precepts, and a higher and better manhood. "Let the medical profession awaken to the fact that it owes a duty to the world more important than simply modifying the results of disease. Moral vices are plunging the nations of the earth into crimes far worse in their effects, present and ultimate, than scores of the diseases for which we have remedies."

Turning from cattle to the "horse," we see even greater evidences of improvement, as the result of care in reproduction. · Here, we see special qualities brought to the highest degree of perfection, independent of instruction in an individual instance. It is noticable, however, that with the higher blooded "horse," his intellectual nature is keeping pace with every other development. The statute, style, action, durability and gait have all been subservient to care in pedigree until the most sanguine expectations of the horseman have been realized. In the dog, intelligence and all those attributes which constitute the desired qualities of its class are brought, so nearly, to a state of perfection that multitudes often express amazement, at the possibilities in dog creation.

Looking now, to the beauties of nature, as seen in the Flower Kingdom, we are told of wondrous changes, and added beauties, brought about through the agency of man, adding up, in certain directions, individual differencies, producing, wondrous and striking changes in their attractive qualities, as well as modifying their aromas to the utmost pleasing degree. And thus we see that man can bring about almost any change he may desire in domestic animals and plants by a careful painstaking study of differencies. Perfection has been the high ideal, and as a result a better product has been secured. Is there less reason, for improvement in the higher order of creation than in the lower, that causes absolute abandoment or neglect of laws, which shall maintain the present standard, or give us an improved class of beings? It is well understood that continued cultivation of a certain soil or of a certain class, without infusing something that shall maintain its power of reproduction, tends to a weaker and lower order of things. This principle and knowledge, is taken advantage of, by man in caring for the lower order of creation, but not his own species. This neglect, along these lines, in betterment of self, is not, as we have seen, in consequence of lack of intelligence and knowledge, of what can be accomplished by "Natural Selection," but, must be the result of neglect, or an uncertain starting point—a sacrifice of high ideals, for mercenary or passionate fancies. I cannot better express my convictions along this line of thought, perhaps, than by quoting the lines of an original thinker, one whose thoughts, although not popular with some, will yet be handed down as among the best, purest and containing more of honest conviction than those of some possessed of more popular favor, one who was born a hundred years too soon. I refer to lines from Robert G. Ingersol: "For thousands of years men and women have been trying to reform the world. They have created Gods and Devils, Heavens and Hells; they have written sacred books, performed miracles, built cathedrals and dungeons; they crowned and uncrowned Kings and Queens; they tormented and imprisoned, flayed alive and burned; they have preached and prayed; they have tried promises and threats; they have coaxed and persuaded; they have exhorted and taught, and in countless ways have endeavored to make people honest, temperate, industrious and virtuous; they have built Hospitals and Asylums, Universities and Schools, and seem to have done their best to make mankind better and happier, and yet they have not succeeded. Why have the reformers failed? I will tell you why. Ignorance, poverty and vice are populating the world. The gutter is a nursery. People unable even to support themselves fill the tenements, the huts and the hovels with children. They depend on the Lord, on luck and charity. They are not intelligent enough to think about consequences or to feel responsibility. At the same time they do not want children, because a child is a curse, a curse to them and to itself. The babe is not welcome, because it is a burden. These unwelcome children fill the jails and prisons, the asylums and hospitals, and they crowd the scaffolds. A few are rescued by chance or charity, but the great majority are failures. They become viscious, ferocious. They live by fraud and violence, and bequeath their vices to their children. Against this inundation of vice the forces of reform are helpless, and and charity itself becomes an unconscious promoter of crime.

"Failure seems to be the trademark of nature, why? Nature has no design, no intelligence. Nature produces without intention, and destroys without thought. Man has a little intelligence, and he should use it. Intelligence is the only lever capable of raising mankind.

"The real question is, can we prevent the ignorant, the poor, the viscious from filling the world with their children? Must the world forever remain the victim of ignorant passion? Can the world be civilized to that degree, that consequences will be taken into consideration by all? Why should men and women have children that they cannot take care of, children that are burdens and curses? Why? Because they have more passion than intelligence, more passion than conscience, more passion than reason. You cannot reform these people with tracts and talk. You cannot reform these people with preach and creed. Passion is, and always has been, deaf. These weapons of reform are substantially useless. Criminals, tramps, beggars and failures are increasing every day. The prisons, jails, poor-houses and asylums are crowded. Religion is helpless. Law can punish, but it can neither reform criminals nor prevent crime. The tide of vice is rising. The war that is now being wagged against the forces of evil is as hopeless as the battle of the fireflies against the darkness of night. There is but one hope. Ignorance, poverty and vice must stop populating the world. This cannot be done by moral suasion. This cannot be done by talk or example. This cannot be done by religion, or by law, by priest or hangman. This cannot be done by force, physical or moral. To accomplish this there is but one way. Science must make woman the owner, the mistress of herself. Science, the only possible savior of mankind, must put it in the power of woman to decide for herself whether she will or will not become the mother. This is the solution of the whole question. This frees woman. The babes that are born then will be welcome. They will be clasped by glad hands to happy breasts. They will fill homes with light and joy. Men and women who believe that slaves are purer, truer than the free, who believe that fear is a safer guide than knowledge that only those are really good who obey the commands of others, and that ignorance is the soil in which the perfect perfumed flower of virtue grows, will with protesting hands hide their shocked faces. Men and women who think that light is the enemy of virtue, that purity dwells in darkness, that it is dangerous for human beings to know themselves and the facts in nature that affect their well-being, will be horrified at the thought of making intelligence the master of passion. But I look forward to the time when men and women, by reason of their knowledge of consequences, of the morality born of intelligence, will refuse to perpetuate disease and pain, will refuse to fill the world with failures. When that time comes, the prison walls will fall, the dungeons will be flooded with light, and the shadow of the scaffold will cease to curse the earth. Poverty and crime will be childless. The withered hands of want will not be stretched for alms. They will be dust. The whole world will be intelligent, virtuous and free. It is far better to be free, to leave the forts and barricades of fear, to stand erect and face the future with a smile. It is far better to give yourself sometimes to negligence, to drift with wave and tide, with the blind forces of the world, to think and dream, to forget the chains and limitations of this breathing life, to forget purpose and object, to lounge in the picture gallery of the brain, to feel once more the clasps and kisses of the past, to bring life's morning back, to see again the forms and faces of the dead, to paint fair pictures for the coming years, to forget old gods, then promises, and threats, to feel within your veins life's joyous streams and hear the martial music, the rhythmic beating of your fearless heart. And then to rouse yourself to do all useful things, to reach with thought and deed the ideal in your brain, to give your fancies wing that they, like chemist bees, may find arts nectar in the weeds of common things; to look with trained and steady eyes for facts, to find the subtle threads that join the distant with the now, to increase knowledge, to take burdens from the weak, to develop the brain, to defend the right, to make a palace for the soul."

In these lines we observe how keenly is appreciated a degenerative tendency under existing comprehension. Intelligence must supplant passion, fancy and fortune. And how shall that be accomplished, is the great and absorbing question. Education along physical lines must be the most potent factor in effecting desired changes. This education will devolve upon the medical profession largely or, at least, primarily, until the principles are more perfectly comprehended in the home. The National Government can, and should do much in bringing about desired reforms, by sending into every home literature, giving wholesome information. Material industries are fostered and abetted by government investigation and experiment. Ignorance, is often more at fault than perverseness or negligence on matters pertaining to reproduction. Improper marriages between the weak mentally or physically or the vicious and criminal classes, should be interdicted by law. With the marriage license should go the endorsement of competent medical authority, after being furnished with authentic family history. With care in these directions, happiness would, in no way, be lessened, but insured as nearly as is possible, other things being favorable. It may seem to many, that such an arrangement, is purely idealistic, and so it may be, but capable of realization if sufficiently and properly agitated by the medical profession, who have a better opportunity of observing the needs of reform than any other class of citizens. By care along these lines, actuated by honest convictions, shrinking not from "Public Opinion," much can be accomplished for the welfare of peoples and nations. It will be truly said that already some states have moved along these lines, and in that much, be it to their credit. The essential need is, that such safe-guards be widespread, numbering all the states and territories, making it impossible to step out of one domain into another to commit an act, which, in their own, is considered unlawful. Strength, force, morality and intelligence, come only from good breeding. A Nation's durability, its dignity and position of influence, depend upon its people and her institutions, all of which, are the resultant force, of proper regard in reproduction. "Nature is revelation, and the light of truth shines everywhere in the world. The want of faith and refusal to reason of men, interposing, make the shadows. Man is blindfolded by himself."

This matter is not one of sentiment alone, but one of serious fact. A question, which must, sooner or later, awaken a lively consideration. It is so far-reaching in its effects, with the pernicious results deseminated, that the superficial thinker, might readily fail to observe its tendencies and ultimate results. Like the wearing of the waters of Niagara upon the rock, slowly but certainly, cutting into and destroying the original stability of society and government. So long as such subjects as Mulligan McNulty, a four term convict of Kansas, who slashed the throat of deputy warden Thomson, from simply a desire, to cut some one, and without provocation, can, at sometime when free, marry and probably be the father of a son, very likely to be born with perverse, if not vicious passions, we cannot hope to lessen our prisons and almshouses, or add to the safety of individuals or institutions. This class of individuals, together with those of mental unsoundness, should be isolated and prevented from marrying, even though they might secure the flower of society. With a proper quarantine, vice and degeneracy could be stamped out, and in its place, liberty, strength and happiness spring up, which would characterize such a condition as that of the millenium. The restrictions and limitations which this paper would imply do not so much refer to the higher order of society, although even this class is not free from violations of such observations in mating as shall secure healthy, sound offsprings. The lower classes contain most of depravity and disregard in the most flagrant manner all conscientious scruples, even carrying known communicable infirmities to the innocent. This class the world over has been the most prolific in populating the world, and sowing the seeds that have occasioned the great demand for prisons, almshouses and asylums. This class has well-nigh taken the management of corporations out of the hands of the owners, and practically disfranchised the sober, thoughtful citizen. The prosperity of a country has never been found to depend upon its great numbers, but upon its intelligence, physical, mental and moral soundness. The principle of expansion which now prevails is undoubtedly good, viewed from a commercial standpoint, but when we look beyond, we might reasonably speculate in regard to the resulting population generations hence. True, we might say, that is a question so remote that we need spend no time in its consideration. But are we correct in discharging this question so peremptorily?

Let us look back but a few years and observe what the feeling has been in regard to unrestricted emigration. A halt has been called, not from lack of domain, but from a lively realization of a too rapid increase of an undesirable element. And so we have every reason to expect might be the result of an extensive aggregation of an inferior people marrying and inter-marrying, without restriction or regulation.· Such has been the history of other countries from which we should profit. Finally not to be interminable, we are impelled to say that degeneracy is the result of fostering or permitting the perpetutation of weakness, moral, mental or physical, each generation growing weaker. *Shall we not waken to the fact and check it?*

DIPHTHERIA AND MEMBRANOUS CROUP.*
By J. W. Lane, M. D., Linneus, Kas.

In the rearing of children, of all things to be dreaded, first is death and next is diphtheria and membranous croup. To the aged, maimed and incurable, death is a source of great relief, but when a disease spreads over the country with a fatality of from 60 to 80 per cent of all the children it is simply appalling. Diphtheria is a specific infectious disease. Characterized by a local fibrinous exudation usually upon a mucus membrane and by constitutional symptoms of various intensity. Early in the disease it may be difficult to distinguish diphtheria from follicular tonsilitis. If the ulcerative process is combined to the tonsils and the follicals stand out bold and prominent it is folicular tonsilitis. If however, it extends to the pillars of the fauces and if laryngeal symptoms develop all doubts are removed and we have a clear case of diphtheria.

The presence of the Klebs-Loeffler bacillus may be regarded as the etiological criterion by which true diphtheria may be distinguished from other forms of pseudomembranous inflammation. Between diphtheria, laryngitis and croup a majority of the writers hold that there is no essential difference; but it is more rational to believe that there is a now specific pseudomembranous laryngitis and I claim that croup is an entire distinct disease from diphtheria. In diphtheria, however, there is almost invariably exudation upon the tonsils or soft palate, while in the nonspecific affection it generally begins in the

* Read before the Grand River Medical Society at Laclede, Mo., Dec. 7th, 1899.

larynx and the fauces are but slightly, if at all affected. It is *not* infectious, for other children stand around and administer to the wants òf the little sufferer and there is not even a thought of contagion. Nor is it followed by paralyisis which is so common in diphtheria, and there is nearly always a suppression of urine.

It is a remarkable fact that while other contagious diseases have diminished, diphtheria, especially in cities, has increased. It has prevailed with great severity in small towns and in the country where the drainage has been imperfect, as dampness always tends to produce sore throat. Among children diphtheria is a highly contagious disease. The poison is given off in the pharyngeal secretion and in the saliva, but not in the breath. If the mucus is coughed out on the clothing, it may be carried to others, or flies may carry it from one mouth to another. Yet it may not be widely diffused in the neighborhood of the patient. Very young children are rarely attacked. The large majority of the cases occur from the age of three to twelve, and more boys than girls are affected. The Klebs-Loeffler bacillus appears to be the specific virus. Both streptococci and staphylococci are frequently found in the exudate; but why spend time in writing on the pathology of this disease for every practitioner is as familiar with the pathology and treachery of diphtheria as he is with the cunning and audacity of a mother-in-law.

In the morbid anatomy I have seen the exudation occur in the mouth and cover the inner surface of the cheeks. Usually the tonsils and pillars of the fauces are both swollen and covered with false membrane. The membrane is of gray color and in extreme cases the parts have a gangrenous appearance. The inflammation may pass into the posterior naris, obstructing the respiration, causing an acid and fetid discharge and a very offensive breath. Extension of the inflammation downwards into the larynx is by far the most serious complication of the disease. It is particularly dangerous in children because it produces what is known as diphtheritic croup. Renal complications are common and nephritis may begin quite early in the disease.

Of the sequela of diphtheria paralysis is the most important, and the greatest to be dreaded is paralysis of the heart, and this may occur at the height of the disease, but very frequently the fatal collapse comes on during convalescence.

Prognosis is favorable if seen in the early stages and treated according to the modern methods. Treatment.—All cases of diphtheria should be excluded from other children. I always instruct the nurse to slip on an old waist before swabbing or spraying the throat, so as to keep the particles of mucus, which are so frequently coughed up, from sticking to the clothing and thus prevent communicating it to other children. Thorough cleanliness, moist air, and good ventilation are three essential points. Thoroughly evacuate the bowels by the free administration of olive oil in hot whisky, calomel or a saline. The throat and mouth must be carefully examined and sprayed every time after giving medicine and no drinks should be allowed for twenty minutes after mopping or spraying the throat, for the drink will dilute and wash the medicine from the affected parts. In diphtheria, if the case is a severe one, I use antitoxin, two thousand units and if necessary follow in twelve to twenty-four hours with one thousand to fifteen hundred units. (P. D| & Co.,) Usually swab the throat every four hours with solution of nitrate of silver, twenty grains to the ounce, and spray throat every hour to an hour and a half with proxide of hydrogen or diphtherine full strength, or diluted one-half, as the case may require. If the case is seen in the first stage and the heart is good, I give aconite and belladona for twenty-four hours, then give per chloride of iron, quinine if indicated. Support heart with strychnia and whisky and give supporting diet.

In nearly all cases of membranous laryngitis there is more or less suppression of urine, in which case I always give balsam of copabia and inhalations from slacking lime, and in nearly all cases the little sufferer will be greatly relieved before through with the first inhalation. I usually first give antitoxin, and then put a piece of unslacked lime in a bowl and sprinkle on it some hot water, place the bowl in a paper sack, place the top of the sack around the child's nose and mouth and let it inhale the steam. If the child objects to the use of the lime I give chloral hydrate to produce relaxation and sleep. This is a much better way to administer lime than making a tent of sheets and much smaller quantities can be used with better results.

In concluding this paper I wish to report a few cases showing some of the complications of diphtheria and the now contagion of croup.

Case I.—Mary S., aged 11. Throat presented all the conditons of diphtheria, membrane covering tonsils and extending upon pillars. Child was sitting up and in fact, never took to her bed on account of sickness. Sent medicine a few days and lost sight of case for about ten days, at which time I was hurriedly summoned and on reaching the house found the child dead, and leaving a history, that for two days previous on attempting to swallow a part of the liquid would return through the nose. This was a case of paralysis of the heart during convalescence, and death was so sudden that she died with her clothes on. Three other children of the same family had diphtheria.

Case II.—Boy aged 5. Did not see case until third day after the attack. Had only passed water once, and twice in twenty-four hours since taken. Great distress was shown in breathing, brazen cough with stridulous, noisy respiration until the whole lower thoracic cavity was drawn in with each inspiration. The eyes were staring and the whole countenance put on that anxious expression which nothing but croup can produce. Cyanosis was very marked both in the hands and face. Gave one-fifth tablet of calomel every hour for five hours. Gave 2000 units of antitoxin (P. D. & Co.) ten drops of balsam copabia every hour and almost constant inhalations of steam from slacking lime as above described. Membrane loosened and was coughed up in exactly twenty-four hours from first treatment. With bowels and kidneys acting freely, child made a rapid recovery and no other children of the family had croup or diphtheria.

Case III.—Boy aged 4½; presented all the characteristics of true croup, and presented all the symptoms of case No. II., with the exception of throwing himself violently when the spasm of the larynx would almost shut off his breathing. Parents would not allow antitoxin used, and I promptly treated him as No. II., with exception of antitoxin, and before he had inhaled the steam from the lime he was breathing, three minutes greatly to the joy of the parents, the delight of myself and to the relief of the little sufferer he was breathing comparatively easy. After the first inhalation he was determined not to inhale the steam. I quickly gave chloral hydrate to produce relaxation and sleep, and continued steam from the slacking lime. Child made a good recovery and none of the children had croup or diphtheria.

Case IV.—Lola T., aged 20, had been treated with domestic remedies and on mopping throat roughly a severe hemorrhage set up. Found tonsils and pillars covered with membrane which extended well over soft pallate and right cheek. Bloody water was exuding from both nostrils and the breath very offensive. Throat and glands greatly swollen and throat gangrenous with every indication of deep seated inflammation, showing the presence of both streptococcus and stophytococcus. Pulse 140 and very feeble and patient showed great exhaustion. Gave one ounce of olive oil, antitoxin, perchloride of iron, quinine and strychnia. Gently touched tonsils with solution of nitrate of silver, XXX grains to the ounce, every four hours, and sprayed nose and throat every hour with full strength proxide of hydrogen. In twelve hours the membrane had all cleaned off and patient made a slow recovery.

QUINALGEN. (ANALGEN.)

BY A. M. WILSON, A. M., M. D.

Professor of Physiology, University Medical College; Professor Materia Medica, Western Dental College, Kansas City, Mo.

Synthetic chemistry has done much for modern therapeutics in the furnishing of medicinal agents of definite character and positive action. Until the laboratories devoted to the production of synthetic remedies begun their physiological experiments and demonstrated their usefulness and reliability. I used very few remedies outside the limits of those found among the alkaloids and similar active principles, because of the unreliability of the ordinary galenicals as found in the drug stores. But now, we have not a few synthetics that are of very great value, and that deserve a permanent place in the U. S. Pharmacopœia, among these Quinalgen takes a prominent position and deserves more than a passing notice.

It has been a hope, long deferred, that some genuine substitute for quinine could be found, something that would possess all the antiperiodic, antimiasmatic and antineuralgic properties of quinine without any of its untoward effects. In fact, a drug that could completly fill the place now held by quinine; and go a step beyond, in also possessing analgesic properties combined with those of a sedative to the nervous system.

Such a drug is Quinalgen—and more—for it is not a mere substitute for quinine in malaria and allied conditions, but seems to reach the very centers of both the circulatory and nervous systems in a most peculiar manner. Under its influence the red blood corpuscles are increased in number and in oxygen carrying power, while both the heart and arteries are strengthened as is manifested by a stronger beat and firmer pulse. On the nerve centres this drug acts as a calmative or sedative where there is irritation caused by morbid matter in the blood, such as we find in rheumatism, gout, lithemia and certain forms of malaria. It does not seem to be of any value in neurasthenia or melancholia or similar disturbances of the mind and nervous system. But in chorea, the nervous depression or mental weakness following some cases of typhoid fever, grippe and cerebro-spinal meningitis, it will be found invaluable, as it not only calms the nerves but also seems to furnish them with a pabulum which disease has removed or impaired. My use of the drug has been confined to the treatment of asthma, chorea, rheumatism and various malarial conditons both acute and chronic, in all of which it has proved itself to be a valuable addition to our materia medica. The malarial cases in which I have tried Quinalgen have been chiefly those wherein quinine has either failed or could not be tolerated because of its untoward effects, such as deafness, severe tinnitus aurium, urticaria and gastro-intestinal irritation.

Mr. Mc., an engineer on one of our railroads has been a victim of malaria for several years. He had run the gamut of all the remedies prescribed for chills and fever, lumbago and the chronic malarial poisoning shown by constant headache, anemia, general lassitude, etc., etc., often having to lay off

*Written for the Index-Lancet.

a trip or two to rest and "brace up," as he termed it. He could not take quinine even in the minutest doses. Arsenic acted fairly well, but neither remedy gave relief, he was placed on Quinalgen, 15 grains every 4 hours for a week, then 10 grains every 4 hours for another week followed by 5 grains 4 times daily for two weeks, when the remedy was stopped for two weeks and again taken in the 5 grain doses for another 2 weeks when it was stopped altogether. More than a year has elapsed since the last dose was taken, but there has been no recurrence of the disease and the man has remained perfectly free from any symptoms of its return.

Miss H., aged 24, neurotic temperment, gave a history of "chills and fever" at intervals of every 3 or 4 months for the past eight years, quinine, iron, arsenic, tonics, Excelsior Springs and visits to other sections of the country had all been tried, but without avail, when she came under my care she looked like a wax image, was listless, no appetite, and did not seem to care whether she lived or died. She said she could not take either quinine or arsenic as they made her worse. I tried both and proved her statement true, for they were rank poison to her though she did not know I was giving them. (I dispense all my own medicine and never let a patient know what is being given.) The quinine caused an intolerable itching and universal erythema followed by extreme prostration, bordering close on to collapse, while the arsenic set up such severe gastro-intestinal irritation that the remedy became worse than the disease.

In this case 15 grain doses of Quinalgen was given every 4 hours for two weeks, accompanied by iron, quassin and strychnia as tonics and appetizers. A complete recovery occurred in the two weeks and no return of the malaria in any form is apprehended as almost a year has elapsed since the case was discharged cured. Many other cases of less severity and occuring in persons ranging in age from 2 years to 70 years could be cited, but the two mentioned are enough to prove the worth of the agent used. It might be well to state that the usual headaches, neuralgic pains, insomnia, general nervousness and debility of long continued malarial poisoning were all relieved by the one medicine. Of course the bowels must be kept regular and all the emunctories in good condition. As is well known gonorrhœal rheumatism is a most stubborn disease to cure, and the more remote from the original cause you see the case the more difficult is the successful treatment. Mr. C. was sent to me by a mutual friend. He gave a history of an illness that simulated inflammatory rheumatism, and for which he had been treated for several weeks some three or four months previous, but received no benefit, being unable to work at his business as salesman in a store. When I first saw him he was pale, anemic, scarcely able to walk, and complaining of great pain and stiffness of both knee joints, and continual pain under the ball of the great toe of the right foot. I was not satisfied with the diagnosis of his previous physician, so said to him,"How long is it since you had gonorrhœa?" He answered, "Who told you I ever had that disease?" I said no one, but I am sure you must have had it sometime before your rheumatism showed itself. He then confessed that he had the "clap" and still had a slight oozing every morning when he first got up. As mentioned before this patient had not been able to work for more than three months, but in one week from the day he began taking Quinalgen he resumed his place in the store and has not lost an hour since. I gave him one dram daily in doses of 10 grains each for the first week, then reduced it to 30 grains daily for two weeks, since when he has been taking 5 grains every 4 hours. Two months has now elapsed since he began treatment and he has had no symptoms of a return of the pain, stiffness or other unpleasant features of the disease. The gleety discharge ceased under the use of calcium sulphide, 10 grains daily.

Several other cases of gonorrhœal rheumatism have been successfully treated with Quinalgen, but none of them were as severe as that of Mr. C.

Mr. P., aged 38, by occupation a bookkeeper, was attacked suddenly with acute articular rheumatism of one elbow joint,, the pain was intense, the inflammation and swelling very great. He was placed on Quinalgen, 5 grain doses every hour for 12 hours, the first 3 capsules containing in each 1 grain of codeine, but after the 3 grains of codeine were taken no other medicine was used except the Quinalgen. When 60 grains had been taken the capsules were given 2 hours apart for 12 hours, then 3 hours between each dose. The pain and swelling gradually lessened until the third day when he was comparatively easy, and on the fifth day was able to be up and dress himself. On the seventh day he could have resumed work if I had allowed him to.

In the above case the temperature ran up to 104° F. and the pain was so severe that one walking across the floor so jarred the bed as to make him scream out. Aside from the 3 grains of codeine, Quinalgen was the only drug used.

Many cases of neuralgic headache, dumb ague, so called sun pain or brow ague have yielded readily to Quinalgen.

But one real test of Quinalgen has been made in treating asthma and that was in a lady 65 years of age, who has suffered with bronchial asthma for more than 20 years, the slightest exertion, excitement or cold bringing on a violent paroxysm of cough, dyspnœa and palpitation of the heart. Aspidospermine, glonon and atropine had always given complete temporary relief, but no remedy had ever been of any continued value until she was placed on Quinalgen, 5 grains every 3 hours, since which time she has had no paroxysms of asthmatic breathing or dyspnœa, though she has passed through the most severe mental and physical strain of her life, and declares that she has never had such a continued spell of comfort for the past 20 years as she has enjoyed since taking this drug. Of course, one case does not prove much, but it is cited for what it is worth.

In the treatment of chorea I am sure Quinalgen will soon take rank above arsenic, as this new drug has a mild but powerful influence on the etological factors in the nervous system, quieting, sedating, and apparently removing morbid material. The most pronounced case of chorea in which Quinalgen was used, was in a boy 9 years of age, who had had cerebro-spinal meningitis two years previous. The choreiac movements were almost constant, especially of the head and lower limbs, occasionally the boy would have a "spell" very closely resembling an epileptic fit. But to make a long story short, he was taken off Fowler's solution, and all other treatment, and given from 30 to 60 grains of Quinalgen daily for six weeks, when all symptoms of chorea had disappeared and the case was discharged cured.

It must be borne in mind that in all the cases referred to, as well as the others not mentioned, the general health of the patients was attended to by such concomitant medicines as seemed indicated in each particular instance. All the Quinalgen I have used was bought in the open market at regular prices and dispensed by myself so that I am certain that no specialy prepared sample was palmed off on me by a manufacturer of chemicals. No toxic or untoward symptoms have thus far been observed as a result of using this agent, no matter how large, frequent or long continued was the dose. The chemical name of Quinalgen (or Analgen, as it is termed in Germany), is ortho-ethyoxy-anamano-benzoye-amido-quinaline. Benzolgen. The dose is from 5 to 15 grains in powder, capsule or tablet. In physical appearance it resembles quinine somewhat, it is slightly sour—not acid—to the taste, is insoluble in water, but freely so in dilute mineral acids and carbonated waters. Its physiological action is that of a non-toxic, antiperiodic, antirheumatic, antipyretic and analgesic, cerebro-spinal sedative and sympathetic nerve stimulant.

THE X-RAYS AS AN AID IN THE DIAGNOSIS OF TUBERCULOSIS OF THE LUNG.

BY J· N. SCOTT, M. D.,
Professor of Electro-Therapeutics, University Medical College.

It has often been said that the most important step in the cure of many diseases, is their early ·recognition. This certainly applies to tuberculosis of the lung. In order to make out the detail of shadows cast by consolidation in the lung by means of the X-Ray, an apparatus which will generate a large quantity of ray, is necessary: but it does not take a very large penetrating power, as the lungs are easily penetrated. If a ray of high penetrating power is used, the darkened areas can not be seen. The penetrating power of the ray can be made so great that the ribs can scarcely be distinguished. What we want, is a ray, just powerful enough to penetrate the normal lung, and not to penetrate the consolidated parts, but make them appear as dark shadows on the screen. The more volume of ray we have with a suitable penetrating power, the more distinct all shadows will appear. We must be able to adjust our penetrating power according to the thickness of the person. The power of penetration of a Crooke's tube is governed by the vacuum. When the vacuum is high, the penetration is great, but lowers as we decrease the vacuum. The volume of ray given by the tube is governed by the volume of current passed through the tube. In order to obtain a large volume of current, I have joined two 12-inch spark induction coils together.

In diseases of the lung, it is much more satisfactory to examine the patient with the fluroscope than to make a radiograph. In all other conditions it is more satisfactory to make a radiograph. A radiograph is often of great assistance in lung trouble, in connection with the fluroscopic examination

A very useful instrument in fluroscopic examination is the Skiameter, devised by Dr. W. Crane. This instrument is made by fastening strips of tin-foil, one c. m. wide, upon cloth covered pasteboard. Six strips are laid side by side parallel with each other, seperated by equal spaces of one c. m. The first strip consists of one layer of tin-foil, the second strip, of two layers, the third, of three layers, the fourth of four layers, the fifth of five layers, and the sixth, one layer, and an equal space below the last layer of tin-foil a metal rod is placed.

I have made up one instrument exactly according to Dr. Crane's direction, and one with strips ¼ inch wide, and spaces ¾ inch wide. If the skiameter is held before the fluroscope, we will see a series of partial shadows of graduated densities. With this instrument we can compare the density of the two lungs, and of different parts of the same lung. It also makes a very convenient instrument to measure the motion of the diaphram.

In an examination of the normal lung by the X-Ray, we find the lung much more transparent on inspiration than on expiration; the ribs are easily defined and an evenly clear light is visible between them. The heart and ascending aorta are easily distinguished. The motion of the diaphram is easily seen. The average motion of the diaphram is about two and one-half inches.

In the beginning of tuberculosis of the lung where there is slight infilteration, it appears as a haziness, and there is not the distinct light appearance of the opposite side, and often on full inspiration the haziness disappears.

If the consolidation is more marked, it may obscure the clavical on the affected side its limits are more marked and sharply defined when changes have taken taken place on one side only, and is easy to compare with the corresponding part on the other side. When both sides are involved, we can tell which side has made the most progress. When comparing both sides of the body, it is absolutely necessary to have the center of the body next the tube, directly in front of the annode, as otherwise distortion will be produced in the shadows. A better view of the apex is obtained from behind, than in front. The shoulders should be brought well forward, thus getting more room between the scapula. The eyes should never be removed from the fluroscope when comparing two sides. It is very important with each examination to measure the movement of the diaphram. When softening takes place, we get a mottled appearance of the affected part, with light and dark spots, also dark streaks. When a cavity is formed we get a light spot surrounded by a dark ring, shading off either to normal lung tissue or consolidated portions.

In many other diseases of the lung we have changes which are shown by the fluroscope. In pleurisy with effusion there is a black shadow extending as high as the effusion, which changes its level with the position of the patient. The lung near the fluid will appear darker on account of the compression. In pneumonia the consolidations cast a shadow on the screen. In emphysema the lungs appear unnaturally clear. In the normal lung, during a full inspiration, the lungs appear much more clear than at expiration. In case we have a thoracic aneurism, a very dense shadow will be thrown on the screen. The shadow is much more dense than that of a tubercular deposit. It will even obscure bone. It is not to be supposed that this method will take the place of the other methods of diagnosis, but it is certainly an aid, and can be used as soon as any consolidation takes place.

---

*REMARKS ON CHOREA, ITS PATHOLOGY AND TREATMENT.

BY JOHN PUNTON, M. D., KANSAS CITY, MO.

Professor of Nervous Diseases, University Medical College.   EDITOR INDEX-LANCET.

LECTURE XX.

Gentlemen:

The subject which I desire to present for your consideration to-day, viz., Chorea, is so common and threadworn that I hesitate to tax your time and patience. Nevertheless various views and opinions are constantly being presented for our approval to account for its varied phenomena, which have both a general as well as special significance that they appeal not only to the knowledge and judgment of the neurologist, but also the general practitioner.

The desire to introduce and promulgate novel and original ideas in regard to disease has become of late so very prevalent and widespread that there is a strong tendency in our day to ignore almost entirely the more common diseases, together with their more settled facts, and substitute in their stead something apparently new and novel, even if it be ever so far-fetched and radical, besides extremely abstract in a vain attempt to satisfy this modern illogical yearning for something extraordinary in subjects medical.

In view of this is it any wonder that I hesitate to invite your attention to so common a theme as Chorea? The physician who poses as a teacher in an up-to-date medical college and presents for his theme such a familiar affection, besides finding himself unable to advance anything strikingly new and original concerning it is liable to be branded as an out-of-date, non-progressive physician, and at best an old fogy. Yet, after all, gentlemen, what can be said of Chorea that is really new and original, at the same time practically benefical since the day when Sydenham wrote his masterly essay?

*Being the substance of a lecture before Senior Class University Medical College.

That the medical world has been asked at varying intervals to accept all kinds of doctrine in regard to the nature and character of Chorea, no one will deny. But how many of these theories have been supported by scientific truth and experience? Yet nothing short of this is worthy our consideration. For instance, in the voluminous annals of medical literature where can be found a more conspicuous series of conflicting theories than those advanced by different writers in their explanation of the pathologic changes said to occur in Chorea. If we turn to our latest text books we find no two authors exactly alike in their findings and the uncertainty which has ever existed concerning its true pathology still remains in spite of the fine spun theories and eloquent warblings of the would-be scientist. Now what is true of Chorea in this direction is also to some degree, at least, true of many other of the more common neuroses. In the universal chase therefore, for something new and novel, let us never despise facts because they are old or allow ourselves to be carried away with the modern craze of apparent pseudo-devotion to science, at the expense of our more rational knowledge. In making this statement I trust I will not be construed as opposing scientific research and experiment or be branded as a pessimist—far from this—for every progressive physician should be also optomistic in his dealing, especially to those that take opposite views from himself. But I desire to emphasize that until we are in possession of positive facts, emanating from reliable sources regarding the true nature of the pathology of even so common a malady as Chorea, our treatment must necessarily be faulty and disappointing and the claims made from time to time by the literary pathologists and advertising schemers for its specific cure by certain drugs based on a false pathology are unworthy the attention of the members of our exalted profession. To-day all the authorities agree that the real pathology of Chorea is unknown, therefore we are practically living in the age of Sydenham, for he admitted this fact and if the statements of our modern reliable authors can be accepted according to them it still remains a mystery. To attempt to enumerate all the theories that have been advanced regarding the pathologic nature of Chorea would be a useless task. Those, however, that are now claiming attention may be divided into three classes, viz.: (1) The Rheumatic. (2) The Neurotic. (3) The Infectious. Each of these have their own special advocates.

The relation of Rheumatism to Chorea is so well recognized that very few deny its presence, and this relation as computed by various authorities varies from 20 to 50 per cent.

The Neurotic theory is based on the constant presence of symptoms referable to their nervous orign as well as complications due solely to Neural involvement. The theory of Infection is perhaps the latest and consequently the most popular. According to this view Chorea is due to a specific germ and by many rheumatism is regarded as an infectious disease, hence its common relation to Chorea is held as a positive proof of its infectious origin.

The Embolic theory of Kirkes is no longer tenable, hence its mere mention is all that is necessary. In the progress of medical science the microscope has played a conspicuous part in unravelling the secrets of tissue metamorphosis and the rubicon which separates organic from functional disease is rapidly disappearing. This in turn has enlarged the fields of pathology, etiology, symptomatology, diagnosis, prognosis and treatment.

In the study of Chorea, however, so far the aid of the microscope has been somewhat limited, but a close observation of its etiology and symptomatology has led to a finer discrimination in diagnosis, and a more scientific classification of its various forms and this perhaps constitutes the chief advance of late which belongs to its specific study. Under the term Chorea, therefore, various spasmodic disorders are now recognized. The most common of all the varieties is that known as Sydenhams chorea which represents the affection, that is ordinarily meant, when the term chorea or St. Vitus dance is used. In order to emphasize some facts concerning chorea I present you this case which is a good illustration of Sydenhams chorea, commonly known as St. Vitus dance.

This young lady patient is 14 years old and I learn that she had a similar attack to the one you now see she has about two years ago. The present attack commenced three months ago during which time she has been under the ordinary arsenic treatment without any special result. About a week ago she came under my observation and in the course of my examination I discovered that she was suffering from heart complication in the form of mitral insufficiency, probably due to endocarditis, which she contracted during her first attack. There is no history of rheumatism, and as already remarked I simply use this case in order to illustrate more forcibly some remarks which are to follow. The affection she is suffering from forms about one-fifth of the nervous diseases common to children, and it usually occurs between the ages of 5 and 15. It is a subacute disorder, characterized, as you see, by irregular jerking and incoordinate movements. Females are more prone to it than males in the ration of about 3 to 1. It occurs in all climates and all seasons of the year. Its causes are both predisposing and exciting, the chief of which, in my experience, are hereditary influences and fright. Injuries and acute disorders, more especially rheumatism, are said to be a potent cause by many authors, but the cases which have come to the University Medical College clinic, as well as my private practice, all demonstrate the fact that rheumatism and its causative agents are a greatly overestimated cause of chorea in children; and in this opinion I find I am not alone. In an article by Dr. Rockwell, of New York *Medical Record* of August 3, 1895, he says: "Notwithstanding all the investigations of and the statistics offered by those who have written upon this subject, I have been unable to satisfy myself that between rheumatism or endocarditis and chorea there exists any constantly direct relation as cause and effect." This view eminently coincides with my experience.

There are many reasons why this is so, and, in my judgment, one of the strongest which he alludes to is the fact that females are more prone to the disease-than males, and yet boys are far more subject to rheumatism than girls. Again, if rheumatism is the cause of chorea, through the action of its toxic agent or its sequel endocarditis, then this should precede the chorea, but experience proves that endocarditis precedes chorea only in a very small proportion of cases.

As a matter of fact, heart disease as a cause of chorea in my practice is comparatively limited, but it is more often found as a sequellæ. By far the greater number of cases that come under my observation are victims of a neuropathic heredity, and this in my judgment is the more potent predisposing cause of chorea, and fright added to this completes its inauguration. One feature that should be emphasized is that chorea having once occurred is apt to occur again and again and the careless habit of trying to quiet the alarm of both the patient and parent as to its serious character by telling them that "it is harmless," and "don't amount to much," and "the child will outgrow it," beside other similar false statements should receive the condemnation it richly deserves for this at best savors of ignorance and incompetency.

Chorea is often found associated with other diseased conditions hence we find it complicating hysteria, rheumatism, epilepsy, insanity, heart-disease, and other acute and chronic disorders. Rarely it is found to exist in the early months of pregnancy, and more frequently as an accompaniment of old age. In most of these cases it manifests itself somewhat differently from the ordinary type, and this fact has led to a more or less imperfect classification, based on the conditions it complicates. Hence we have senile chorea, hysterical chorea, maniacal chorea, the chorea of pregnancy, etc.

Moreover, in view of the fact that it is sometimes localized, another class is recognized under the term "convulsive tics," or unilateral chorea. Commenting on this, Dana says: "There are many persons who go through life with some trick of speech or gesture, or some peculiar grimace. It may be a shrug of the shoulder of a twitching of the eye or nodding of the head, but they all represent abortive attacks of chorea, and are usually embraced under the term 'habit chorea,.'"

Procursive or dancing chorea is, according to Laycock, characterized by spasmodic rhythmical contractions, or by sudden rotating or procursive movements of the body, when the condition of the patient is similar to that of a person who has been whirling round a number of times. This form of chorea is usually associated with hysteria.

The term "electric chorea" was first applied by Dubini to a progressively fatal spasmodic affection observed by him solely in Italy. It is really an aggravated and violent form of the ordinary Sydenham chorea.

But of all the rare and interesting forms of chorea none are more serious and fatal than hereditary chorea. This disease was first accurately described by Dr. Huntington, a Long Island physician, in 1872, and it is now often termed Huntington's chorea. The disease rarely begins before the 30th or after the 50th year, and is almost always due to hereditary influences. It begins without any known cause, by twitching of the muscles of the face which gradually extends until it involves the whole organism. It is a chronic progressive disease, accompanied by both physical and mental deterioration, with a tendency to melancholia, and finally ends in dementia and death. The muscular movements are entirely different from those of the ordinary Sydenham type. For instance, in Huntington's chorea, the muscular movements are of far larger range and whole groups of muscles are simultaneously set in motion. The disease therefore is never a localized one. The speech is frequently altered and there is more or less impairment of the mental faculties, while the curaneous sensibility is rarely altered, but the patellar reflexes are usually exaggerated. As the disease progresses, the patient may become entirely helpless, and the dementia may also become absolute.

The pathology of this form of chorea, like that of Sydenham's, is still unknown, and its prognosis is always exceedingly grave, because a case has never been cured. It is comparatively rare, and for this reason I am induced to report the following case. which recently came to my clinic; besides, it beautifully illustrates its hereditary nature, and many other interesting facts regarding its peculiar character.

J. J. C., aged 36, male, white, telegraph operator, a native of Bohemia, single, first came under my observation August 25, 1895, and gave the following history: His ancestry shows that his mother died in an insane asylum. while his father enjoyed good health. There were seven children, four of whom are dead; one died of cholera, two from cramp colic, and one from the same disease that my patient now has—viz., hereditary chorea. He has one sister. who married a drunkard and who abused her so that she lost her mind, and she is now confined in the Topeka Asylum.

At the age of 23 the patient states that he contracted syphilis, but went under treatment at once, and believes he fully recovered from it. On stripping him. there was no external evidence of its presence. His habits were not of the best. although he says he never drank to excess, but smoked a great deal. About five years ago. when he was 31 years of age. he found the muscles of his face began to twitch like he used to see those of his brother. This gradually increased and progressed until it involved all four extremities, and for the last two and one-half years it has entirely incapacitated him from all kinds of work.

The patient was greatly reduced in flesh and more or less anemic. The peculiar muscular movements were very marked and almost incessant. They were of wide range, and it seemed as if the whole muscular system .twitched in groups simultaneously. In walking the patient presented marked inco-ordination, besides making all kinds of strange gestures, which attracted the attention of the public. Cutaneous sensibility was unimpaired, but the patellar reflexes were exaggerated. The voice was somewhat high-pitched, and he spoke with a nasal twang. His memory was gradually becoming impaired, and there was marked deterioration. The patient was unable to assign any cause for his trouble, unless it was his work as a telegraph operator.

He had consulted several physicians, and everything they had done for him proved unavailing, as there was a steady, progressive, bodily and mental decline. All kinds of diagnoses had been made, according to his own state-ments, by the different doctors, such as locomotor ataxia, paralysis agitans, multiple sclerosis, alcoholic neuritis, etc., which finally had the effect of shak-ing his faith in the efficacy of the science of medicine, and he had decided to abandon all hope of getting any assistance from physicians, when his fellow-telegraph operators, moved by sympathy in his behalf, raised a fund and in-sisted on his making a further trial, and sent him to me. The same uncer-tainty which characterized the diagnosis also pertained to the prognosis, some advising a high altitude and others a low one; a few thought a tropical climate would be best, and others declared this would be fatal to him; while occasionally he was assured by apparently good physicians that they could cure him. Such statements, however, should meet with the censure they richly deserve, when we remember that so far no case of cure has been reported.

I might say that I am inclined to believe that we are all disposed to re-gard the subject of chorea as a trifling matter, and, because of its common occurence and general character, treat it with indifference. No disease, in my judgment, is more prone to be attended with more serious sequelae, when improperly managed, than chorea; and for this, if for no other reason, it demands the earnest attention and painstaking care of every medical practi-tioner that undertakes to treat it.

Treatment:—From what has already been said any plan of treatment we may adopt must necessarily be more or less speculative.

On general principles, however, there are two things that the major-ity of physicians believe are indicated in the treatment of chorea: 1st, rest, and 2nd, the administration of arsenic. Of the two, rest is by far the most important and generally the more complete the rest the speedier the cure. Choreal children, therefore, should be taken from school and the parents instructed to put them to bed and keep them there for a vary-ing length of time. The more severe the chorea the more urgent the need of absolute rest in bed. To secure the full benefit of this measure the patient should be protected from all sources of excitement not even being allowed to associate with accustomed playmates, but the isolation should be complete.

The medicinal treatment of chorea is unsatisfactory. With the excep-tion of arsenic no remedy seems to have any special influence in control-ing the progress of the affection. Even this, at times, is unavailing. To augment its efficiency, however, many drugs are employed, but their specific effects are very limited. For some time I have been using the medicinal preparation commonly known as arsenauro with the very best of results. As its name implies, it is a combination of gold and arsenic, and was first brought to the attention of the medical profession by Dr. Barclay under the name of liquor auri et arsenii Bromidi.

Its use in my practice has been attended with better results than any

other single remedy in this affection.   In addition to arsenauro other tonic
remedies, such as iron, quinine, cod liver oil, malt and similar drugs in
combination with mild sedatives such as the various preparations of the
bromides or small doses of hyoscyamus, cimicifuga, cannabis Indica are
sometimes beneficial at different stages of the affection; many other drugs however are recommended by different writers for its relief.   But to sum
up the treatment of chorea in a few words, I think that rest and freedom
from all sorts of excitement, combined with tonics and careful attention
to the diet, is the most rational of all prescriptions.

EXTRACTS AND ABSTRACTS.

*SPLANCHNOPTOSIS.

Some general remarks upon the subject of Ptosis of the Abdominal Viscera by Albert I.
Bouffleur, M. D., of Chicago.

It would be discourteous even to my sense of propriety, did I not avail myself of this, my first opportunity of expressing to the members of the Academy
my appreciation of the honor conveyed by your cordial invitation to address
you upon this occasion.   After consultation with your President I have chosen
as the subject for my necessarily brief remarks, "Ptosis, or dropping down of
the Abdominal Viscera."
The attention of the profession was first called to this condition by Glenard, who was evidently quite carried away by the etiological importance of
the condition to which he had given much thought.   Various observers have
since given the subject consideration, and have added many valuable contri-
butions to the literature thereof.   In fact, the subject has been so amplified,
and the observations and reports have been so numerous that it will be impossible for me to treat the subject, or even any single phase of it with a satisfactory degree of exhaustiveness, in the time at my disposal.   I will, therefore,
limit my remarks to a few general statements upon the more common phases of
abdominal visceroptosis.   The term enteroptosis was employed by Glenard to
indicate a prolapse of the stomach and intestines with the occasional involvement of the right kidney, etc., which gave rise to various neurasthenic and
dyspeptic symptoms.   There has seemed to be a tendency on the part of some
writers to continue the use of the term to indicate general ptosis, but in view
of the fact that each organ now forms the subject of extensive observations, we
believe it would be more accurate and scientific to follow the suggestion of
Stiller and designate ptosis of two or more viscera as Splanchnoptosis, or pos-
sibly Visceroptosis, and indicate the displacement of the individual organs by
their anatomic names: e. g. gastroptosis, nephroptosis, enteroptosis, hepatopto-
sis, etc.   While prolapse of the pelvic viscera might with propriety be considered a part of this subject, since they are in many respects dependent upon
the same causes, etc., they present certain special features which seem to war-
rant their separate consideration.
Varieties.—The condition may be congenital as suggested by Stiller, and
as demonstrated by the absence of the normal attachments of the organ involved, or it may be acquired.   The latter is the more common variety.
Causes.—There seem to be two principle factors in the causation of
splanchoptosis: viz.:

*Abstract read before the Kansas City Academy of Medicine

1. Weakness of the attachments or normal means of suspension, and
2. Diminished abdominal pressure or support.

Traumatism, either direct or indirect may cause displacement of organs. A direct blow to the loin in the lumbar region has caused the loosening of many kidneys, while jumping from heights and falls have been given as exciting causes by many patients. Excessive weight of an organ, as by tumor formation—or dilatation and overdistention as observed in a dilated stomach, or an overloaded, constipated colon would naturally be causes for displacement. Any chronic wasting disease, which would cause a weakening of the ligaments and supporting attachments of an organ, or which would cause the absorption of fat (e. g. tuberculosis, chlorosis, hysteria, dyspepsia, etc.) would deserve recognition as a cause of visceroptosis. The remarkable frequency with which this condition is observed in thin, pale, weak, dyspeptic, neurasthenic men and women demonstrates beyond successful contradiction the influence of this factor. Another element in the production of attenuation and weakening of the supports is that of pressure when applied from above as by a pleuritic effusion or a dilated stomach, or when applied, from the sides as by tight lacing or the improper suspension of clothes, or by a combination of the two as by overlifting. There can be no question whatever but that the narrowing of the lower segement of the thoracic cone by persistent firm pressure as produced by tight lacing, or tight waist bands, is productive of disturbed relations and even ptosis. The proper use of corsets is not necessarily productive of displacement, in fact, when intelligently fitted and properly worn they may even support the abdominal organs in their normal positions, thus serving the purpose of a therapeutic measure. The effect of the strap or belt as worn by some men about the waist has a similar effect to tight waist bands and is a fruitful course of enteroptosis.

The second causative factor noted was diminished abnormal support. The abdominal wall forms the sides of a cavity with more or less flexible walls. As the cavity is for practical purposes filled with fluids in which various organs are suspended, it stands to reason that anything which diminishes the resisting properties of the walls, modifies the position of the organs, as does also variations in their comparative specific gravities. The two conditions most likely to cause relaxation of the abdominal walls are overdistention, as by repeated pregnancies, tumor formations, etc., and the position or carriage of the body. Attenuation of the abdominal wall is under some circumstances a physiological performance of heavy work would naturally interfere with normal involution, and as the organs would thereby be deprived of their normal counter pressure, their displacement would be the logical result. The person who commonly assumes a stooped or flexed position in sitting and thereby relaxes the abdominal muscles, encourages the development of atony and attenuation of the abdominal wall. This is particularly noticeable in those who do not indulge in active exercise, and when they are in an erect position, depend upon their process and involution, usually takes place to a marked degree. Early rising after parturition, improper support, lack of corrective exercise and the early stays for maintenance of the erect position. As there are so many conditions which may logically cause ptosis of some viscera, it does not require much imagination to formulate the natural sequence of events which might occur in a given case.

The tranverse colon is so frequently overdistended that from weight alone it would naturally descend, and in doing so traction would be made on the pylorus, causing some obstruction to the escape of stomach contents which would collect and by weight cause gastroptosis. These by pressure would cause discent of the small intestines and the resulting indigestion and malassimilation would naturally result in malnutrition of all the structures of the body, and after a while the kidney and liver supports would be weakened and the intra-abdominal presure so diminished that prolapse of several of the organs would be the logical result. Likewise, in an individual of delicate constitution, naturally thin and anaemic, with poor digestive and reconstructive powers, we do not find any tissues of the body in a robust, healthy condition, and in these when the fossa retaining the kidney is usually shallow, a slight indirect traumatism might result in a displacement of the kidney, which in time by traction upon the duodeunum or bile ducts would cause disturbance of the function of those organs, etc.

Frequency.—Meinert reports having found some degree of gastroptosis in 80 per cent of 14 year old girls, and some form of abdominal ptosis in 90 per cent of his private female patients, and 5 per cent of male patients. Einhorn reports having detected some form of ptosis in 13 out of 33 females complaining of stomach troubles. ·As to the relative frequency of ptosis of the different organs, we must place the right kidney first. It occurs perhaps in 20 per cent of female patients, and its relative frequency as compared with the left is perhaps best explained by the shallowness of the paravertebral fossa on the right side, as seems to have been conclusively demonstrated by the experiments of Wolkow and Delitizien; 2nd, the colon; 3rd, the small intestines; 4th, the stomach; 5th, the left kidney; 6th, the spleen; 7th, the liver, etc.

Symptomatology.—The symptomatology varies greatly; some cases of slight ptosis cause severe and even alarming symptoms, while other cases of even marked displacement are unproductive of symptoms. As Treves has stated, there are;

1. Cases of splanchnoptosis which present no subjective symptoms.

2. Cases of even moderate degree of ptosis which are attended by distressing and even alarming symptoms of a purely nervous character, and

3. Cases of ptosis causing mechanical disturbances which are productive of typical symptoms. To the second class we can with propriety give the name of Glenard's Disease, since these present the phenomena he reported so graphically to the profession. This class of cases occurs in the thin, anaemic, poorly nourished individuals, whose minds and nervous systems are in a condition of starvation. In a general way these patients become depressed and are in poor health. They tire easily and are liable to fainting spells and cardiac and aortic palpitation, and usually present symptoms of indigestion. Their appetite fails, sensation of weight and distress after eating is present, and nausea and vomiting may occur. They complain of all varieties of nervous symptoms and particularly of headache and insomnia. The bowels are irregular and usually constipated. Laxatives cause distress. These symptoms are aggravated and frequently occur only when the erect posture is assumed. The organ displaced will naturally be productive of special symptoms directed to the system involved, e. g., Nephroptosis is frequently productive of renal colic and other symptoms of hydronephrosis, while displacement of the liver may cause jaundice, etc.

Diagnosis:—Splanchnoptosis occurs most frequently in thin, weak, neurasthenic persons. A flat abdomen is usually associated with neurasthenic symptoms. Those presenting a pendulos abdomen are, according to Mathieu, usually free from them. The upper part of the abdomen is flat, even hollowed, while the lower quadrants are bulging. The aorta is quite invariably readily detected. The position of the stomach and colon can be demonstrated by inflation, etc. The position of the liver and kidney and other organs in general, can be determined by palpation and percussion which, however, must be made with the patient relaxed in the inclined or vertical position. Palpation of movable kidneys, which is frequently impossible in the recumbent posture, even with the assistance of inspiration may be successful with the patient in an over vertical position. Glenard laid great stress upon the diagnostic value of pressure applied to the lower part of the abdomen by means of the hands of the physician, who should stand behind the patient. The relief afforded was frequently marked. Stiller believed that the 10th rib is always abnormally movement in these cases, and as it would indicate a fibrous attachment of that rib, it would give weight to the argument that this condition is one of faulty development, as he claimed.

Treatment:—The treatment of abdominal visceroptosis must necessarily vary with the degree of the ptosis, the resultant effects and the surrounding circumstances. It may properly be divided into palliative and curative.

The palliative treatment consists 1, in the maintenance of the position conducive to the restoration of the affected organ to its normal position. 2. In the encouragement of the fat forming properties of the organs. 3. In the systematic use of massage to restore the tonicity and support of the abdominal wall, and, 4, in the wearing of a properly fitting supporter.

The value of massage and gymnastic exercises is generally underestimated in the treating of this class of cases. The employment of inflated rubber bags as advised by Futterer, for the retention of a floating kidney is frequently most gratifying in its effects. As curative measures, the foregoing are of but little value except massage and physical cultures which by restoring the abdominal wall to its normal condition will undoubtedly frequently relieve all the distressing symptoms presented. The curative measures are essentially operative in character. Treves advises simple abdominal section as a curative procedure in those cases occurring in the thin, neurasthenic class which are so prolific in the production of disturbances of the nervous system.

The results of this procedure in his hands would seem to indicate that the effects are largely psychological in character, and by relieving them, the condition itself is placed with these not productive of any symptoms. This would seem to be an entirely too roseate position to take, since the general health of the patient is in such cases always far below normal and must need careful attention, while the presence of the ptosis would render the reproduction of the original symptoms more than likely. As an adjunct in the treatment of such cases the simple exploratory incision undoubtedly has its place, but as a curative procedure for genuine ptosis we fail to appreciate its application. Treves has anticipated such opposition by classing the operative effects with those in tubercular peritonitis, etc., in which the clinical value of the procedure must be recognized, even though we may be unable to explain its modus operandi.

The operative procedures of most value are splanchnorrhappy which is essentially an anchoring of the viscus and splanchnectomy, which implies the removal of the offending organ. The employment of the modern technique in the operation of nephrorrhaphy has proved so satisfactory that it would seem to be indicated in practically all cases of nephroptosis giving rise to symptoms. Palliative measures should be tried in cases presenting contra-indications to immediate operative measures, but their use should be only temporary, unless perchance, they render the patient perfectly comfortable and restore her to health. Anchoring the liver has been attempted a few times, and from a recent experience in this line I am fully convinced that it is a practicable operation and when the technique is more perfectly developed it will be quite as satisfactory as nephrorrhaphy. Floating spleens have been successfully anchored with satisfactory results. Enterorrhaphy and gastrorrhaphy, which con-sist essentially in reefing the mesentery and the lesser omentum respec-tively, have not been sufficiently employed to enable one to speak as pos-itively of their curative value as in anchoring of the more solid viscera, but the results have in general been encouraging. While by reefing we may restore the organ to its normal position and by applying the proced-ure to the walls themselves, the size of the organ may be reduced, the pathological changes in these organs will necessitate a course of medical treatment and a guarded prognosis. Removal of an organ for ptosis must of necessity be indicated very rarely. Nephrectomy has been re-sorted to a number of times, but the possible absence of the fellow kid-ney, the higher mortality of the procedure and the satisfactory results of the present method of nephromtophy has placed it as an extremely rare method of treatment in this condition.

Splenectomy has been resorted to a number of times, and fully half the authorities consider it a safer and better operative proceedure than splenorrhaphy. This may be true in those cases of marked floating spleen in which the function of the organ has been repeatedly interrupted, but in displacements of a moderate degree there would seem to be no valid excuse for depriving the body of an organ, concerning the physiological value of which we are so ignorant.

In addition to anchoring and removal of the affected organs, various plastic procedures have been advised for the relief of ptosis. The for-mation of the peritoneal pouch as devised by Pean representing one type, while the resection of the abdominal wall as advised and successfully practiced in two cases by De Page represents the extreme degree to which some operators have gone in attempting to devise methods productive of uniformly satisfactory results. While the operative technique must nec-essarily vary somewhat with the different organs, owing to their varied nature and anatomical surroundings, it would seem to be a fact that an-choring of a displaced organ is the simplest, safest, most rational and satisfactory manner of treating that condition. While the methods of examination as to the position of the solid viscera have been so perfected as to admit of ready employment and the diagnosis of ptosis of those or-gans has, therefore, become more frequent, the investigation as to the position and condition of the hollow viscera has not become a general practice, and until the method of diagnosis are improved, these cases will probably be generally considered as marked cases of Dyspepsia as hereto-fore.

The more frequent diagnosis of nephroptosis has resulted in an ap-parently satisfactory technique for the anchoring of that organ, and I have no doubt but that the methods of operating for ptosis if the other organs will be so improved and perfected as to give equally satisfactory results. I would, therefore, admonish you to make more careful exam-inations of this class of cases with the patient in proper position there-for, and am confident that you will be surprised at the frequency of the presence of some form of splanchnoptosis, and I believe you will find the above suggestions as to treatment generally satisfactory.

In addition to the corrective measures, I would like to briefly call your attention to the preventive treatment of this condition. There is certainly no class of disease in which the old adage "an ounce of preven-tion is worth a pound of cure," is more applicable than in this condition. It is much easier to assist a weakened support than to restore one entirely destroyed, and likewise, it is easier to prevent loss of abdominal sup-port than to restore it. As prophylatic measures I will mention:

  *1. Correct carriage and position of the body, which of itself is preventive of the pendent abdomen now becoming so common with American men and women.

2. Correct arrangement of dress, particularly in the young and adolescent, and after the operation of any of the causes enumerated.

3. Maintenance of muscular tonicity by massage and systematic exercises; this is especially advisable in those who supplant their muscles by stays for a great portion of the time. The daily employment of proper treatment would obviate much of the harm of such a practice, and lastly,

4. The proper support of the abdominal wall after unusual or prolonged distention and after prolonged illness.

The responsibility of the physician should not cease with the recovery from the immediate malady under treatment, as by proper advice we may often make our patients stronger men and women than they were before a serious illness. Our efforts should always be directed to securing the restoration to normal of the whole body, and not merely the single organ whose trouble caused our employment. While this subject is yet in the early stage of development, and our knowledge is more or less fragmentary, it is constantly growing and with more observations and experiences, there is every reason to believe that the obscurity of the causes and effects of this medley of manifestations will be elucidated and that its treatment will be correspondingly satisfactory.

FROM HOSPITAL RECORDS OF CASES TREATED BY TROPHON-INE MEDICATION AT METRPOLITAN HOSPITAL,
BLACKWELL'S ISLAND, N. Y.

L. C., age 28, native of Ireland, occupation, domestic.

Diagnosis:—Extreme anæmia, following the puerperal fever (incipient phthisis).

Family History:—Unknown; previous history nothing of any value obtainable.

Present History—About two months ago patient gave birth to a living child, her first pregnancy. After confinement was sick for some time with puerperal fever; now suffers from extreme pain in abdomen. Has offensive vaginal discharge, abdomen very sensitive and tympanitic. Patient runs a typical hectic temperature, has severe night sweats. Has a constant and weakening diarrhœa.

Subjective Symptoms:—Patient is very weak, unable to move, great pain in abdomen when moving; short of breath on the least exertion.

Physical Examination:—Pale, waxy, emaciated and covered with perspiration; general emaciation.

Circulation:—Anæmic murmers at every cardiac orifice. Bruitde-diable heard with great distinctness in jugular veins. Size of heart normal. Has enteric involuntary diarrhœa.

Respiration:—Dullness, both apices as far down as the first rib on the right and second left. Bronchicial breathing and an increased vocal fremitus. Crepitant rales heard at apices.

Genito-urinary System on Dec. 12th:—Patient was placed before a clinic as an example of anæmia; the murmers were pronounced. Patient was unable to stand up during examination.

Treatment:—Patient was placed on two tablespoonfuls of Trophonine, to which was added two drops of Guaiacol and two drops of Creosote. This was given every four hours. Her condition rapidly improved, the color returned to the cheeks and patient was soon able to be up and about. The same treatment was continued for the next three weeks, but as additional treatment, two Protonuclein Special Tablets, two hours before meals and before retiring were ordered. Within five weeks after admission into the hospital, patient was discharged as cured.

COMMUNICATION.

CUBA, KANSAS.

TO THE EDITOR OF THE KANSAS CITY INDEX-LANCET.

DEAR SIR:—I would like to present to INDEX-LANCET an idea concerning the location of the lobular pneumonia, and pulmonary tuberculosis. To me it seems very plausible, and has been partially verified in all the cases of tuberculosis that have come under my observation since the idea first occurred to me.

Lobular pneumonia is given by authorities as most frequently located in the lower right lobe, and pulmonary phthisis in the right apex in the beginning. The size and direction of the right bronchus favors the turning of a greater amount of bacteria to the right, than to the left lung. But the bronchial tubes are not apparently arranged to separate the *pneumococcus* from the *bacillus tuberculosis*. The difference in the circulation of the base and apex of the lung is held by some as the cause of the difference of the location of these two diseases. Now, I offer the *position during sleep* as an important condition affecting the difference in the circulation, so as to render the right apex more susceptible to attack by the tubercle bacillus.

Most persons sleep on the right side with the right arm drawn forward and toward the anterior median line of the body, with the forearm flexed and the hand under the face, and the body inclined *venter* downward. This position from pressure impedes the circulation of the right apex and limits its respiratory motion. The tubercle bacillus is able to gain lodgment here. but is resisted by the more active circulation and respiratory motion of other parts of the lung, and by this part, except when impeded.

Now the pneumococci, as well as tubercle bacilli, are usually breathed into the lungs when one is in the upright position, and the greater number of each, and all, probably go to the base of the right lung. Here or in any part of the lungs the pneumococci are able to overcome the resistance of the tissues, provided other causative factors of pneumonia are present. It is the position during sleep that I present as an important cause of tuberculosis beginning in the apices of the lungs.

Of eleven cases observed, as a student and later a practitioner, seven were of the right and four of the left apex. Of the seven all say that they slept on the right side at the time questioned or before contracting the disease. Of the the four, three say they slept on the left side and one on the right.

I would be glad to hear this reported on, from one having the advantage of a larger observation.   Very truly,

W. F. HOWARD, A. B., M. D.

FOR SALE CHEAP.

A first-class general practice for sale cheap in the suburbs of Kansas City. House, lot 75x120, office fixtures, with good will. Annual income, $4,000. Apply to the Editor, Index Lancet.

PHYSICIANS ON ISLANDS.

The startling fact was recently made public that, in many districts of Puerto Rico, where the population reaches thousands, there is no resident physician. For instance, Wayuya, a town of 1,500, must depend upon the simplest remedies in the case of illness, as there is no physician within call. At Utuado, the death rate is 8 per cent annually, and this town is a day's ride from Ponce through the mountains.

It appears that physicians have been sent to these districts, but they refuse to remain, largely because no town is able to support one. As a result of this condition of things, the order providing a physician for every 500 people is now very difficult of enforcement, because the towns reply that there is no fund for such service.

This island is one vast poorhouse, and there are opportunities for charity at every step.

Were $10,000 to be expended immediately for medicine and medical aid, it would possibly save the lives of 3,000 people. At one time the government considered the feasibility of assigning a physician to each town, at an aggregate cost of $80,000 per year, but the funds for such an outlay are not available.

OBITUARY.

Dr. Alfred Baxter Sloan died April 17th, at his home in Kansas City. On account of poor health Dr. Sloan had not been practicing medicine for several years. Recently he suffered an attack of pneumonia, which was the direct cause of death.

Dr. Sloan came to Kansas City in 1865 and for many years was prominent in his profession in Kansas City. He was one of the founders of the Kansas City Medical Society, of which he was president for twelve years; a member of the Jackson County Medical Society; once treasurer and vice-president of the of the American Medical Association and a member of the International Medi-Missouri State Medical association; for six years one of the judicial council of the American Medical association and a member of the International Medical Congress, which was held at Washington in 1887.

Dr. Sloan's early life was pent on farms in Lafayette and Jackson counties. He received his school education at Lexington, Independence and Rich Hill, Mo. He studied medicine under Dr. Joseph C. Boggs of Independence, brother of L. W. Boggs, a former governor of Missouri. After graduating from the Transylvania University of Kentucky, he began the practice of medicine in Bates county, Mo., in 1848, and a year later he started to the gold fields of California. He returned to Missouri by way of Panama in 1852 and resumed the practice of his profession at Harrisonville, Mo. In 1861 he and Tarlton Railey of Cass county, his father-in-law, started for the Pike's Peak gold region in Colorado, hauling machinery for a quartz mill across the plains from Leavenworth, Kas. Returning home the next year, he joined the Confederate army of General Price at Osceola as a surgeon. He served in the Sixteenth Missouri infantry in Missouri and Arkansas. He was soon promoted to quartermaster of the Confederate army stationed along the Arkansas river, and served in that capacity unti the close of the war, when he came to Kansas City and engaged in the practice of medicine. Dr. I. M. Ridge is the only physician now in Kansas City who was practicing here when Dr. Sloan opened his office.

SOCIETY MEETINGS.

KANSAS CITY ACADEMY OF MEDICINE.

Incorporated under the laws of the State of Missouri, June 28, 1890.

OFFICERS SINCE ITS ORGANIZATION.

H. G. Crowell, M. D., President....1890	C. Lester Hall, M. D., President,....1894
W. C. Tyree, M. D., " 1891	John Punton, M. D., " 1895
B. E. Fryer, M. D., " 1892	John H. Thompson, M. D., " 1896
J. H. Duncan, M. D., " 1893	C. F. Wainwright, M. D., " 1897
Resigned April 25.	Robert T. Sloane, M. D., " 1898
Emory Lanphear, M. D., elected to fill	Hal Foster, A. B., M. D., " 1899
unexpired term.	

OFFICERS FOR 1900.

Jabez N. Jackson, M. D. President; John M. Langsdale, M. D., Vice President; Bennett C. Hyde, A. B., M. D., Censor; Ralph J. Brown, M. D., Secretary; C. Lester Hall, M. D., Treasurer.

MEETING OF APRIL 7.

Dr. Dulin presented a case of Abdominal Aneurism.

CASE 1—Mrs.——, age thirty-two, married fourteen years, housewife, four children the oldest of which is twelve years of age.

Present illness began twelve years ago immediately after birth of first child with pain and throbbing sensation in the epigastrium. Has complained constantly and at irregular intervals has paroxysms of dyspnoea and vertigo. Has been relieved of these attacks by use of cardiac stimulants.

Family History suggests no point of importance.

Previous illnesses ordinary diseases of childhood; typhoid fever eleven years ago. Miscarriage two years ago, the result of uraemia at fourth month of pregnancy. Denies any venerial disease and examination shows no evidence of such.

Examination of patient at intervals of once a week during the past eight months shows the following condition:—Rational, poorly nourished and aenemic. Slight exophthalmus, small bi-lateral bronchocele, aenemic hum over jugulars Pulse irregular. Chest symetrical but retracted supra and infraclavicular Heart rapid and at times irregular. Pulse soft and compressible with exception of temporal arteries. Abdomen flabby, (enteroptosis). Spleen not palpable. Liver dullness normal. Pulsating, expansil tumor reaching from the costal arch to umbilicus immediately to left of vertrebal column, with a bruit and thrill most distinct at a point one inch above and one inch to the left of the umbilicus. The bruit is transmitted to the illiac and femoral artries. Genitalia, limbs and reflexes normal, no adenopathy.

Urine—Sp. G. 1.020 Reaction acid color high albumin, considerable puss none casts, hyaline and granular.

Blood—Haemoglobin 80% Red corpusles 3400000 white corpusles 34000 or one white to 100 reds.

Diagonosis Aneurism of abdominal aorta.

This has been a case of extreme interest first because a young women; second because she had never had syphilis or any chronic disease; third, has lived an easy life and has never had to perform hard labor. None of the commonetiologic factors can be considered in this case, but one of extreme rarity, the extreme muscular exertion necessary to bring on expulsion of first child.

Dr. Fryer read a paper on Gleanings from Pathology in which he spoke on the retrogressive changes in the neuron, the absence of Nisl's chromophil bodies in fever. He thought Cohnheim's theory of tumors was as free from criticisms as any, but that none were absolutely unobjectionable. Serum therapy received a very favorable comment, as did also immunity. Drs. Binnie, Dulin, Hibbard, Cordier and Brown discussed the paper.

MEETING OF APRIL 14.

Dr. Jabez N. Jackson presented some X-ray pictures of a case of exostosis. Case was a young athlete who while playing football had received a slight injury, which at the time seemingly of no importance. Since he had felt a hard growth beneath the skin which seemed to be gradually enlarging. Advised an X-ray to be taken which showed an extosis, and removed the growth.

Dr. Dulin said I wish to simply show you the gross specimen and microscopical preparation, you will notice that the tumor is about the size of a walnut and seems to grow from several centers. It is cartilaginous and is found at the end of a bony pedicle 1½ inches long; evidently enchondroma from a microscopic view, but the unusual feature of this case is revealed by the microscope. The superficile tissue consists of a stratified layer of cubical cells; underlined which are numerous capillaries showing an obliterating endarteritis, with hyperplasia of connective tissue. The deep sections show nothing but typical hyaline cartilage. It is interesting to study this section because stratified epithelium is not found in bursa; there is no explanation for the occurence of epithelial tissues in benign bony or cartilaginous growths; there is no history, symptoms or signs of syphilis, consequently endarteritis is a sign that is hard to explain.

NEW YORK ACADEMY OF MEDICINE. SECTION ON ORTHOPÆDIC SURGERY

Meeting of March 16, 1900.

LENGTHENING THE TENDO ACHILLIS.

Dr. R. A. Hibbs presented five patients affected with talipes equino-varus, the result of infantile paralysis, on whom he had performed a new operation, as follows: The tendo Achillis having been exposed by a parallel incision 1½ inches in length, made to its outer side, it was cut transversely within ½ inch of its insertion; through two-thirds

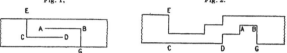

Fig. 1,   Fig. 2.

of its substance, and with the turned knife it was then split upward a certain distance. A quarter of an inch above the end of the longitudinal cut another transverse cut was made from the opposite side through two-thirds of the substance of the tendon and the knife being turned the tendon was again split to within ¼ inch of the first transverse incision. Thus the tendon was severed in such a manner as to secure its lengthening and at the same time to preserve its continuity. In figure 1 the first transverse cut would be from E to C, the first longitudinal from C to D, the second transverse from G to B, and the second longitudinal from B to A. When traction was applied lengthening would occur as shown in figure 2, and it would be equal to the sum of the two longitudinal cuts minus the sum of the two laps of ¼ inch each. In figure 1, if C D is ½ inch; B A ½ inch, A to E C ¼ inch, and D to G B ¼ inch, then the lengthening would be ½ inch plus ½ inch minus ¼ inch plus ¼ inch, or 1 inch minus ½ inch, or ½ inch. It was a matter of choice whether the longitudinal or the transverse cuts were made first, but it was important that the skin incision should be to the outer side of the tendon in order to prevent the scar from falling directly over the tendon, which might be rubbed by the shoe. Dr. Hibbs had learned since operating by this method that it had been practiced in a case of traumatic equinus by Sporon, a Dane. (Hospitalstidende, 3rd series, Vol. IX, No. 50, 1881.)

CASE I.—In a girl eight years old, a short tendo Achillis had prevented flexion of the right foot within 10 degrees from a right angle. It was lengthened by this method on Sept. 22, 1899, and the foot was fixed at a right angle. In two weeks slight voluntary motion was allowed and the muscle received daily exercise with some resistance from the attendant, After ½ inch lengthening had been secured there was positive resistance to any further flexion of the foot than was allowed by the lengthening. The child walked with strong control of the os calcis.

CASE II.—In a girl twelve years old flexion of the left foot was impossible within 15 degrees from a right angle. The tendon was lengthened ¾ inch on July 6, 1899. With suitable after treatment the result was an excellent position of the foot, with strong action of the muscles of the calf.

CASE III.—In a girl fourteen years old flexion of the right foot was prevented within 10 degrees from a right angle. The tendon was lengthened 1¼ inch on June 16, 1899, an unusual amount in order to relieve extreme valgus, with resulting good control of the os calcis. As the valgus was recurring a tendon grafting would be done.

CASE IV.—In a girl eight years old the left foot was inflexible within 45 degrees from a right angle, appearing to be almost in a straight line with the leg. The tendon was lengthened 1¼ inch on June 16, 1899, and the foot fixed at a right angle. It was believed that an ordinary tenotomy would have been followed by loss of usefulness of the calf muscles. It was seen, however, that this action was excellent.

CASE V.—In a girl fourteen years old the right foot had been inflexible within 15 degrees from the right angle and the tendon was lengthened ¾ inch on June 16, 1899, and the foot fixed at 90 degrees. The muscle and tendon showed enough strength to sustain the weight of the body on tip-toe, and this had been true of all the cases presented.

In no case had an effort been made to correct the equinus beyond a right angle. Further correction might be desirable in congenital but not in acquired equinus.

That the strength of a tendon lengthened in this way was not seriously impaired was proved by the observation that in every case there had been resistance to the carrying of the flexion beyond the limit allowed by the operation, and also by the ability of the muscle and tendon to sustain the body on tiptoe   The process of repair had been rapidly completed after operation by this method, which presented obvious advantages over those in which sutures were applied to the tendon.   But the greatest advantage had been found in the readiness and certainty with which the desired amount of lengthening could be exactly secured.

A perfect gait required the "spring" or elastic quality imparted by the muscles which enabled the anterior part of the foot to sustain the weight of the body in walking. Without this power the gait would be that of one who had a wooden foot or a foot affected with talipes calcaneus   In equinus following infantile paralysis it was probable that the muscles were more shortened than the tendon, and, as lengthening the muscle was generally impossible, operative relief had to be sought by lengthening the tendon. In operating, however, it was important on the one hand to avoid leaving the tendon so long as to impair the action of the muscle and on the other hand to avoid leaving it so short that the equinus would not be sufficiently overcome.   This method enabled the operator to maintain exactly the proper relation between the length of the tendon and that of the muscle.   By subcutaneous tenotomy the equinus was readily corrected, but in many cases the result was a serious defect in the gait from undue lengthening of the tendon and resulting shortening and inefficiency of the muscles.

Dr. A. M. Phelps said that it was immaterial whether a muscle was operating at its full length or whether the same amount of muscle tissue was operating at a shorter leverage.   The power was precisely the same, as instanced by putting your arm nearly straight or flexing it.   Open incisions for primary operations on the tendons should be avoided, and in the ordinary subcutaneous operation the tendo Achillis should be made too long if possible by over-correcting, the normal process of repair being relied on to fill in the space between the ends and to secure an accurate and efficient adjustment of the relative lengths of the structures.   He had repeatedly seen 4 inches replaced after division of the tendo Achillis and perfect function of the muscle restored.

Dr. Hibbs said that an alteration in the relative length of the muscle and its tendon modified the effect of muscular contraction.   If the tendo Achillis was lengthened the contractile power of the muscle cells might remain but the extent to which the os calcis could be raised by the contraction of the muscle would be lessened.   If the muscle of the calf could not momentarily sustain the weight of the body on tiptoe in the act of walking they were not of great use.

Dr. H. L. Taylor said the fear of impairment of function after ordinary tenotomy properly done and followed up was unnecessary.   It was formerly the custom after division of the tendon to put the foot up in the deformed position and to correct the deformity at subsequent sittings.   Correcting the deformity immediately after the operation was attended with good results.   It was possible to elongate the tendon too much, but such cases were rare.   He had been looking for years for a case of ununited tendon after tenotomy, but had not found one.   The exact amount of correction would vary with the kind of case.

Dr. H. Gibney said that he had seen one or two adults in whom the tendons had failed to unite.   He could see no advantage in the new operation over the ordinary subcutaneous method; after which many cases acquired a length of 2½ inches.   The results shown, however, were excellent, and would be better still after tenderness and an indisposition to voluntary motion had worn off.

Dr. J. P. Fiske said that the results shown were good, and that the details of the new operation were very interesting.   It was, however, a departure from the rule of simplicity which characterized the old operation which, almost without exception, gave results which left nothing to be desired.

Dr. A. B. Judson said a short tendo Achillis produced no deformity and did not interfere with the normal gait excepting in cases in which the tendon was extremely short.   Normal flexion of the ankle might be said to be about 40 degrees within a right angle, but with 10 degrees the gait was normal in appearance and ability, and the patient experienced no inconvenience, even when assuming the unusual position of squatting.   In measuring the equinus it was desirable to have the leg flexed on the thigh in order to relax the gastrocnemei which had their origin in the femur.   The foot being held flexed manually, so far as it could be done painlsssly, one arm of the goniometer might be made parallel with the crest of the tibia and the other parallel with the inferior surface of the os calcis and the head of the first metatarsal bone.   The degrees could then be read on the scale.   In the use of the club-foot brace for congenital equino-varue setting the upright backward from a right angle lengthened the tendo Achillis, which was contrary to what might have been expected.

Dr. Taylor had a few years ago offered an explanation of this action of the club-foot

BLENNOSTASINE.

GIVES GOOD RESULTS IN ALL FORMS OF CATARRHAL HYPERSECRETION.

"I have used Blennostasine in night sweats of consumptives with great benefit."

"Blennostasine is the best remedy for cold in the head I know of."

"Blennostasine gives instant relief in early stages of cold in the head."

"Blennostasine gives relief in acute cases of rhinitis, but is of little service in chronic cases."

"The more I use Blennostasine the more I am satisfied with it; I have had wonderful results from it."

"I have been surprised at the promptness with which it would relieve the common cold of the nose and throat. I have used it now for over a year."

"I have used Blennostasine with good effect in acute rhinitis."

"I have found Blennostasine the most effective remedy in treating 'grip' and influenza that I have ever tried, and much prefer it to the synthetical drugs."

"There is nothing so far produced that anywhere near equals its action in acute coryzas—colds. A few doses decreases the secretion, relieves the weight and heaviness of the head and the cold can generally be made to dissapear in twenty-four to thirty-six hours. It is a vaso-moter constructor that is non-toxic and certain in its action. It is very gratifing indeed to witness the celerity of its action. It is a permanent improvement in our materia medica."

"Blennostasine in particularly applicable to colds of singers and speakers, as the blednostatic effect is preferable to that of belladonna, and certainly produces a tonic effect on the vocal mechanism."

"I think we have in this drug a very useful remedy for aborting coryzas and acute laryngeal colds, and much prefer it to preparations of belladonna."

EXCERPTS FROM RECENT COMMUNICATIONS.

Samples and Literature Free on Application.

McKesson & Robbins, - New York.

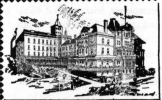

brace by the theory that, as the inner border of the tendo Achillis was shorter than the outer border, when the foot was rotated outward by the brace the inner border was first put on the stretch and gave way, fibre after fibre. thus unexpectedly lengthening the whole tendon.

Dr. Hibbe said that he had operated in this manner on upwards of twenty patients, but those presented had been the only ones in whom sufficient time had elapsed to make the presentation useful. It was vastly more important to preserve the action of the muscles than to relieve the deformity, which was generally not serious and in some cases absent.

· LITERARY NOTES.

Mr. Robert P. Porter, who was Superintendent of the Eleventh Census, and who was sent last year to Cuba and Puerto Rico as special commissioner for the United States to investigate the industrial and commercial conditions prevailing there, has written for the April North American Review a very valuable paper on "Our European Trade"— more especially our trade with France. Germany and Great Britain. The fact of most startling import in the history of our recent commercial development is the vast increase in our exports of manufactured articles, which during the past fourteen years has reached the astounding aggregate of two hundred million dollars. Mr. Porter calls attention to the consternation which has been produced in the minds of some of our European rivals by this unprecedented progress, which signifies the eventual change of the United States from an agricultural and raw-material producing state to an industrial state, although the volume of our agricultural exports has by no means decreased. This extraordinary development Mr. Porter regards as the most conclusive vindication of the wisdom of our protective policy.

"A Missionary in the Great West," by Rev. Cyrus Townsend Brady; "The Choir Boys of England," by Julian Ralph; "The Mysteries of the Century," "Singing 'The Messiah' on the Plains," "Behind the Scenes During a Play," "College Girls' Larks and Pranks," give an idea of the varied excellence of the April Ladies' Home Journal. Of course, Rudyard Kipling's "Just So" story, "The Elephant's Child," narrating with delightful humor how the elephant got his trunk, will be sought first and heartily enjoyed. Ian Maclaren identifies "The Genteel Tramps in Our Churches," Edward Bok points out the evils of "The Ease With Which We Marry," and "An American Mother." writes on "The American Woman in the Market-Place." "Bandanna Ballads," by Miss Howard Weeden, and "Fairies in Funnyland" combine rhythmic and artistic beauties. The first of a series of journeys "Through Picturesque America" fills two pages, and "A Successful Country House in New England" and "Wellesley Girls in the Play" are also pictorial features. A fair part of the April Journal is filled with matters of interest to women. By The Curtis Publishing Company, Philadelphia. One dollar a year; ten cents a copy.

Those who have read the "Tiverton Tales" of Miss Alice Brown will not need to be urged to secure the May "NEW LIPPINCOTT," in which appears her first novel, "April Showers," complete. All the rustic beauty and humor which made up the "Tiverton Tales" are here lavished on a novel whose plot is fresh and new and whose characters are racy of New England life. The tale turns on the theft of a baby by its own reprobate father, the runaway mother having died. There is a counterpart of love; deceit, and manly constancy. For the price of a single magazine one may thus obtain a book more powerful and no less charming than the author's earlier success.

To any reader of the daily newspapers, or in fact, any one who desires to keep abreast of the complicated and rapidly shifting developments of the present day, the monthly magazine CURRENT HISTORY, is a work of exceptional utility. It is admirably clear in style and judicious in treatment, confining itself to summarizing each month the important news of the world, divested of all non-essentials, giving only facts without trying to mould sentiment one way or another, and so conveniently arranged as to form a permanent record eminently worthy of preservation for reference. It is well printed on excellent paper and abundantly illustrated with authentic portraits, maps and views. It combines the features of a cyclopedia of current history, a dictionary of present-day biography, and a portrait gallery of national and international celebrities, with all the freshness and interest of an historical novel. The contents of the April number range from South Africa to the Orient, from Alaska to Australia, from the Philippines to the West Indies and Latin America, and cover all matters interesting the nations in all parts of the world, the progress of Science, Art, Religion, etc.

BOOK REVIEWS.

THE YEAR BOOK OF THE NOSE, THROAT AND EAR. G. P. Head, M. D , and
    and A. H. Andrews, M. D. Chicago Medical Book Co., 1900. Cloth, $1.50 net,
    postpaid.

In the above work the authors have conceived the idea of reviewing the
literature of the nose, throat and ear and have tried to glean the essential points from the leading Journal articles of the year.

The book has 256 pages of valuable reading, 148 devoted to the nose and
throat and 118 to the ear. The articles are more complete than are usually
found. The book is well printed on good paper, and we think this an
excellent idea and trust the authors will continue its publication from
year to year.

THE EXPOSE OF WELTERMERISM. MAGNETIC HEALING DE-MAGNET-
    IZED. By Preston W. Pope, M. D., Nevada, Mo. Price, 65 cents.

In publishing this little volume the author's purpose is to set forth the
leading features of Weltmerism; to point out its errors and their logical
sequence; to indicate the principles and practice of so-called magnetic
healing which are worthy of further study or adoption; to direct attention to the true science of healing, health, happiness and eternal life.
The author is a regular practicing physician of a number of years experience, and has investigated the teaching and practice of these magnetic
healers and gathered from all available sources of medical lore and skill
everything that would prove interesting in this little volume. While it
is but a paper back yet it is very interesting.

PROGRESSIVE MEDICINE. Volume 1, 1900. A quarterly digest of advances, dis-
    coveries and improvements in the medical and surgical sciences Edited by Hobart
    Amory Han, M D., Professor of Therapeutics and Materia Medica in Jefferson Med-
    ical College of Philadelphia. Octavo, handsomely bound in cloth, 404 pages, 36
    engravings and a colored plate. Lea Brothers & Co., Philadelphia and New York.
    Issued quarterly. Price, $10.00 per year.

The scheme of Progressive Medicine as carried out last year has proved
to be so excellent that no material alteration has this year been found
necessary. In a few minor matters some changes have been made, for
instance, greater attention has been paid to therapeutics, prescriptions
have been quoted when necessary, etc. Vol. 1, treating of surgery of the
head, neck and chest—infectious diseases, including acute rheumatism,
croupous pneumonia and influenza—diseases of children, pathology,laryn-
gology and phrenology, otology, Dr. DeCosta's references to diseases of
the mammary glands,and Dr. Packard's careful investigation into serum—
therapy in diphtheria, and his authoritative statement summing up the
consensus of opinion as to the Brand method of treatment in typhoid are
worthy of special note. Dr. Blackader's contribution exhibits the same
painstaking, practical qualities as did the corresponding chapter in the
volume of last year. In fact, the entire contents of the volume will be
found up-to-date and of the utmost value, and will be warmly welcomed
by the profession throughout the entire country.

SCATTERED LEAVES FROM A PHYSICIAN'S DIARY. A series of satirical
    sketches from real life, reflecting more or less upon the men who control it, by Al-
    bert Abrams, A. M., M. D. (Heidelberg) F. R. M. S., San Francisco, author of
    "The Antiseptic Club," etc.; pp. 68, with frontispiece; 50 cents. St. Louis, Mo.
    Fortnightly Press Co., publisher.

MULFORD'S GLYCERINIZED VACCINE

"ALWAYS TAKES"

Furnished in Improved Package Combining Scarifier

NOTE CUT

Literature with photographic reproductions, showing method of preparation and full information, mailed postpaid, upon request.

H. K. MULFORD COMPANY

PHILADELPHIA CHICAGO

Per case of ten vaccinations, with scarifier, case and bulb for expelling Lymph, $1.00 postpaid
Supplied by reliable druggists only

ONLY ONE

**product—food—contains all the elements necessary to restore impoverished blood and wasted tissues.
Only one remedy,**

GRAY'S GLYCERINE TONIC COMP.

assures adequate assimilation of food in anæmia, convalescence and malnutrition.

THE PURDUE FREDERICK CO.,

No. 15 Murray Street, New York.

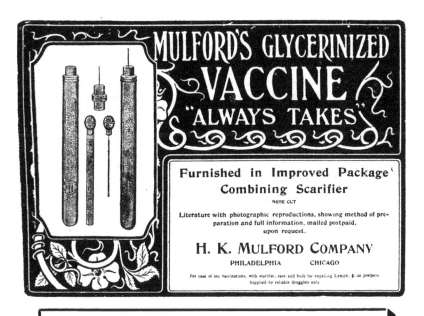

Please mention the Journal when you write to an advertiser.

In this little pamphlet the author places a mirror, as it were, up before the empiric, in which he may be able to see himself as others see him, containing many amusing and entertaining delineations of character illustrating the various methods by which the professional dignity is lowered; revealing, also, human nature as it is met with by the medical fraternity. The pamphlet is of exceeding interest because of its elegant portrayal of the ease with which the people are gulled by the quack, and because of its keen sense of humor therein contained.

HYDE ON THE SKIN. New (5th) edition. A practical treatise on diseases of the skin, for the use of students and practitioners, by James Nevins Hyde, A. M., M. D., Professor of Dermatology and Venereal Diseases in Rush Medical College, Chicago. In one octavo volume of 866 pages, with 111 engravings and 24 full-page plates, 8 of which are colored. Cloth, $4.50 net; leather, $5.50 net.

A work that has reached its fifth edition within such short time needs very little commend to prove its value. The work has been thoroughly revised, material being found of no longer importance has been eliminated and new chapters written or certain subjects, as Porokeratosis and Blastomycetic Dermatitis. Among the subjects that have been wholly or in part revised, are the following: General Etiology, General Therapeutics, Eczema, Pupuia, the Alopecias, the Atrophies, Lupus Erythemalosus, Mycosis, Fungoides, the Neuroses, Xanthonia, Pellagra, Impetigo, Dermatetes Herpetiformis, Pigment anomalies, Tuberculosis, Syphilis and Mycetoma. New illustrations have been furnished by the addition to the text of twelve full-page plates and two engravings. Its value as a student's text book, as well as a work of authority in the profession, will doubtless be more realized in this edition.

HEMMETER ON DISEASES OF THE STOMACH—Their Special Pathology, Diagnosis and Treatment, with sections on Anatomy, Physiology, Chemical and Microscopical Examinations of Stomach Contents, Dietetics, Surgery of the Stomach, etc. By John C. Hemmeter, M. D., Professor in the Medical Department of the University of Maryland, Baltimore. With many original illustrations, a number of which are in colors. Second edition, enlarged and revised. Octavo, 898 pages. Price, $6.00 net. Cloth. P. Blakiston's Son & Co., 1012 Walnut street, Philadelphia, Pa.

The second edition of the work which is practically a re-written book, a great part of it having been reconstructed and a large amount of new material added, of which the following articles are the most important: Hypertrophic stenosis of the pyloris, obstruction of the orifices, the use and abuse of rest and exercise in the treatment of digestive diseases, hemorrhage from stomach. The most useful feature of this second edition is the repeated and thorough application of nature and critical judgment to the entire subject matter of the book. While the text is one which is not sufficiently large to constitute a genuine specialty, yet the volume will furnish the general practitioner valuable assistance from which he can readily acquaint himself with the advances in this important branch of medicine. The book will take a prominent position among the works of its text.

ELEMENTS OF CLINICAL BACTERIOLOGY. For physicians and students. By Dr. Ernst Levy, Professor in the University of Strasburg. i. E.; and Dr. Felix Klemperer, Private Docent in the University of Strasburg, i. E. Second revised and enlarged edition. Authorized translation by Augustus A. Esher, M. D., Professor of Clinical Medicine in the Philadelphia Polyclinic; physician to the Philadelphia Hospital, etc. W. B. Saunders, 925 Walnut street, Philadelphia, 1900. Price, $2.50 net.

This work represents an attempt to group the results of bacteriologic investigation from the clinical point of view, being a translation of a well known work on clinical bacteriology. While the general practitioner is not expected to be a practiced bacteriologist, yet is is well that he be familiar with the subject, and we believe this work is adapted to the present position of bacteriologic knowledge. While the volume is not very profusely illustrated, yet it is sufficiently so as to be of value in this particular point. The work is written in a manner evidently intending it for the general practitioner and covers the bacteriologic situation in a manner which is completeness itself, and is a masterly work on the subject.

GOULD & PYLE'S CYCLOPEDIA OF PRACTICAL MEDICINE AND SURGERY
A concise reference book, alphabetically arranged, of Medicine, Surgery, Obstetrics Materia Medica, Therapeutics, and the various specialties, with particular reference to Diagnosis and Treatment. Compiled under the editorial supervision of George M. Gould, A. M., M. D., editor of ''The Philadelphia Medical Journal,'' etc., and Walter L. Pyle, A. M , M. D.. Assistant Surgeon to Wills Eye Hospital. 73 contributors. Quarto. Illustrated. Sheep or half dark green leather, $10.00; thumb index, $11.00; half Russia, thumb index, $12.00. P. Blakiston's Son & Co., Philadelphia, 1900.

This volume represents the writings of seventy-three contributors of authority, revised, arranged in a concise form, and edited by Gould and Pyle, who are well known by the profession as needing no recommend. They have provided a trustworthy hand-book of easy reference in physical and clinical diagnosis, general therapeutics, operative technique, materia medica, toxicology, and other subjects concerning which information is constantly needed in undergraduate study and in daily practice. Diagnosis and treatment receive particular attention; minor subjects which are of great value to the practitioner, but usually omitted from the textbooks, are here given proper consideration. Under the most common title diseases and inquiries are classified according to the part involved. A frequent recourse to the recent medical periodicals and text-books and the standard medical dictionaries and cyclopedias of all languages make the book up-to-date and a thoroughly reliable reference work or twin companion to Gould's Illustrated Dictionary of Medicine. A uniform system of bold-face headings have been adopted so that the subject matter may be seen at a glance. Printed on good paper and well bound, and should be found in the library of every studious physician.

MISCELLANEOUS,

Dr. Arthur Hulett, of Chicago, Ill., has located in Kansas City.

Dr. Samuel G. Gant and wife, of New York City, were visiting with old friends recently. Dr. Gant is connected with the New York Post Graduate Medical College.

Dr. Fred P. Reed and Miss Elizabeth Norton were married at Weeping Water, Neb., April 18th. Dr. and Mrs. Reed will be at home at Black Hawk, Colo., after May 15. The INDEX-LANCET extends its best wishes for a happy future.

Dr. W. L. Ray, first assistant physician of State Lunatic Asylum No 1, was elected superintendent by the board of managers to fill the vacancy made by the resignation of Dr. J. T. Coombs. Dr. Emil Theilman, second assistant physician, was advanced to first physician, Dr. J. A. Reilly, third assistant, was advanced to second, and Dr. Edward H. Tinchnor of Mexico was the new member of the staff elected by the board to fill the position of third assistant physician.

Pil. Antiseptic Comp.

(W. R. WARNER & Co.)

℞ Sulphite Soda, 1 gr.
Salicylic Acid, 1 gr.
Nux Vomica, ⅛ gr.
Powd. Capsicum, 1-10 gr.
Concentrated Pepsin, 1 gr.

DOSE—1 to 3.

PIL. Antiseptic Comp. is serviceable in atonic dyspepsia, nervous dyspepsia—in fact, all forms of this disease, because it strengthens the lowered digestive vitality

The Nux Vomica and Capsicum, besides promoting involuntary contraction of muscular fibre, relieve flatulence and constipation.

The digestive properties of the Pepsin, assisted by the action of the Salicylic Acid and Sulphite of Sodium, in addition to the above, make this an effective remedy.

Pil. Cascara Cathartic

(W. R. WARNER & Co.)

A SOLUBLE ACTIVE PILL.

℞ EXT. BELLADONNA, ⅛ gr. Peristaltic stimulant to the bowels.

GINGERINE, ¼ gr. To prevent griping and for its carminative properties.

STRYCHNINE, 1-60 gr As a tonic to the intestines.

CASCARIN, ¼ gr. Removes and prevents constipation.

ALOIN, ¼ gr. Increases peristalsis of lower bowel.

PODOPHYLLIN, 1-6 gr. Increases peristalsis of the upper bowel, and mildly stimulates the flow of bile.

Renews Peristalsis.

Relieves Hepatic Torpidity.

Mild in Action.

An Intestinal Tonic.

SPECIFY "WARNER'S."

Pil. Chalybeate.

(W. R. WARNER & Co.)

A Most Satisfactory Method for Prescribing Iron as indicated in

ANEMIA, CHLOROSIS, PHTHISIS.

℞ Ferri Sulph.
Potass. Carb., aa 1¼ grs.
DOSE—1 to 2.

PIL. Chalybeate produces Ferrous Carbonate in the stomach, and mingling with the gastric juices is more quickly assimilated than any other preparation of iron.

Pil. Chalybeate Comp.

The same formula as Pil. Chalybeate with ⅛ gr Nux Vomica added for its tonic effect.

THEY ARE BLOOD MAKERS.

SEE THAT YOU GET NO SUBSTITUTE.

Pil. Arthrosia

(W. R. WARNER & Co.)

℞ Acid Salicylic.	Ext. Phytolacca.
Quinina.	Ext. Colchicum.
Res. Podophyl.	Pv. Capsici.

DOSE—1 to 2.

AN ANTIDOTE FOR

..RHEUMATISM AND GOUT..

PIL. Arthrosia combines pure drugs, accurately subdivided. scientifically compounded, a quickly soluble coating (hermetically sealing and protecting contents indefinitely). Upon administration, Pil. Arthrosia will disintegrate rapidly and release a combination of remedies whose known therapeutic properties at once recommend this pill to the profession.

A marked improvement in rheumatic diseases follows almost immediately after taking Pil. Arthrosia.

W. R. WARNER & CO.,

Philadelphia. New York. Chicago.

The Eighteenth Congress of Internal Medicine opened at Weisbaden, Germany, April 19th.

The late Dr. Axtell has been succeeded by Dr. W. N. Beggs as editor and publisher of the *Colorado Medical Journal.*

Dr. J. M. Minick of Wichita, Dr. J. E. Locke of Holton, and Dr. A. S. Gish of Oberlin, constitute the new members of the State Board of Health.

Dr. John F. Lapp was sent to Butler, Mo., to investigate the small pox condition, and found thirty-two cases. A local quarantine is in effect in four of the smaller towns adjacent to Butler.

The National Academy of Science in Washington, recently awarded the Bernard medal to Wilhelm C. Roentgen, the developer of the X-Ray. This medal is given once in five years to the person making the most important scientific discovery during the period.

Dr. C. B. Simcoe, of St. Joseph, Mo., has been appointed by the governor to be superintendent of the new colony for the feeble-minded, which is to be located at Marshall, Mo. Dr. Simcoe has been an assistant at the St. Joseph Hospital No 2, for the past three years.

Dr. George F. Butler has been appointed Superintendent of the Sanitarium at Alma, Michigan, to succeed Dr. E. S. Pettyjohn, the appointment to take effect May 1st. Dr. Butler will retain his college connection with the Chicago College of Physicians and Surgeons, and will continue to edit the *Doctors' Magazine.*

Mr. J. I. Fellows, 48 Vesey street, New York, has issued a very interesting little pamphlet entitled, "The Test of Time and Experience," in which are graphically described the symptoms and conditions calling for the use of his Syrup of Hypophosphites, together with the results which may be expected from the same.

Dr. S. E. Sheldon of Topeka, died very suddenly April 19, at his home from heart disease. He had practiced as a physician and surgeon in Topeka for thirty years. Dr. Sheldon retired apparently in good health. His wife was later awakened by his struggles, which almost immediately terminated in death. Dr. and Mrs Sheldon had planned to start soon for a trip to Europe.

Dr. J. T. Coombs, the homeopathic physician whom Governor Stephens, three years ago appointed Superintendent of the State Insane Asylum No 1, at Fulton, Mo., has resigned. Ill health is given as the cause. His resignation was one previously tendered by request of the board, as a result of an investigation of charges of drunkeness and immorality, but Governor Stephens refused to accept this resignation.

Six years ago Isaac Smith, country school teacher, near Russiaville, was suddenly bereft of his reason, just on the eve of his marriage to Miss Effie Gossett. The day the ceremony was to have taken place Smith was taken to the state insane asylum at Indianapolis, a raving maniac. Brooding over the affair finally dethroned Mise Gossett's reason, and she was sent to the same asylum, where the demented lovers, unknown to each other, occupied wards for five years. Last week Smith, being fully recovered, returned home. Miss Gossett is rapidly improving, and a permanent cure is expected speedily. The marriage will then be solemnized.

The Secretary of War has forwarded to Congress, with his approval, the draft of a bill prepared by Surgeon General Sternberg providing for the appointment of contract surgeons, who have rendered one year's faithful and satisfactory service in the army of the United States, with the rank of first lieutenant, as assistant surgeons of volunteers.   The bill provides for such appointments after the usual examination as to physical and professional qualifications, and the officers so commissioned are to be subject to honorable discharge whenever their services are no longer required.   The bill also provides for the promotion of such assistant surgeons to the rank of captain after two years' faithful and satisfactory service.

The Cigarette. —Cigarette smoking has become a potent cause of insanity, as shown by statistics from the hospitals and asylums throughout the country. In Chicago the average in one hospital is more than twenty-five cases annually, or 2 per cent of all insane cases.   It is peculiar to this phase of nervouse decadence that the mental ruin is generally too grave to be reparable.   Medical science is incapable of helping these suicides of the mind; and all that remains, as they are generally violent, is to subject them to restraint like incorrigible animals whose physical vigor survives for a time their intellectual death.

Although the effects of cigarette smoking are generally understood, dealers continue to sell the poison without restriction.   The druggist is required to label prussic acid or strychnine or arsenic when he sells any one of them.   The dealer in cigarettes might with equal propriety label his poison if its nature were not as well known.

THERAPEUTIC HINTS.

A late treatment of general septicemia is by hypodermic injections of creosote.   The creosote is mixed with equal parts of camphorated oil, and 20 minims of the solution are injected three times a day.—*N. Y. Med. Times.*

Malarial Toxaemia.—The following method of treatment gave me excellent results in a case of malarial toxæmia with sallow skin, furred tongue, bitter taste, profuse sweats, cough, pain in right shoulder, also pain and tenderness in right hypochondrium and congestion of the liver:
R   Salol,
Quinine sulph., aa dr. ss.
M. et div. caps. No. xij.   Sig.   One every three hours while awake, and the following gien night and morning:
R   Pulv. ipecac, gr. iv.
Ext. colocynth comp., gr. xij.
Mass hydrarg., gr. xxiv.
M. et div. caps . No. xij.   Sig.   One night and morning.—*Medical Summary.*

Gastric Irritability. —In cases of gastric irritability of bottle-fed babies, where there is a frequent eruction of milk after nursing, ingluvin has proved of service.   It will promptly check the diarrhea which is caused by indigestion. By reason of its influence upon the stomach and bowels, it is capable of marked service in cases of cholera infantum.   The dose is from 1 to 2 grains.

Hyoscine Hydrobromate In Chorea.—Hyoscine hydrobromate has been tried by A. C. Rendle, of Madras, India (*Brit Med. Jour.*, No. 2013, 1899), on a bad case of chorea in a youth of 16 years.   He was thin and anemic; the temperature was slightly raised; the tongue was dry and coated with a brown-

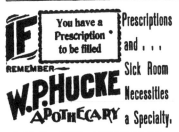

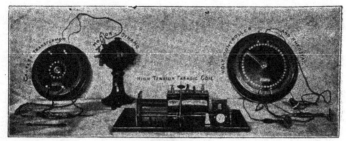

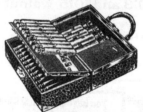

ish fur; the pulse was weak and the respirations irregular; there were constant involuntary movements. Albumin was present in his urine. Potassium bromide, chloral hydrate, and increasing doses of arsenic gave no relief. He was very restless at night, and morphine eased him slightly. Hyoscine hydrobromate in doses of 1.200 of a grain was injected hypodermically twice a day. On the following the first injection there was marked improvement in the choreal movements. The dose was increased to 1.100 of a grain and given three times a day. In a week the movements had almost entirely ceased. The hydrobromate was then discontinued and the arsenic treatment resumed. The patient made an excellent recovery. Chorea is an extremely fatal disease in India.—*Alienist and Neurologist.*

A Case of Sinus.—G. W. Bodey, M. D., of Kettlersville, O., says: "I used Ecthol on a case of sinus extending from the inner and middle of the right thigh upward and outward nine and one-quarter inches in length. It had been operated upon in that locality twice, also once on the canal from the psoas abscess, its starting point. The sinus was lined with a tough pyogenic membrane, so that by inserting the index finger its full length occasioned no pain. The young man twenty-two years old, would submit to no further operation. I inserted perforated rubber tube, one-half inch in diameter, nine inches, burned or destroyed the membrane with chloride of zinc solution, after which I used Ecthol, filled the cavity completely full three times a day, by which the pus ceased to flow from the very beginning. I continued its use until I could not insert even a catheter. I applied a rubber bandage for five weeks, dismissed him then as cured; the period extended eight months. I used five bottles of Ecthol. I dismissed the case in May last, and will wait to see further results, then I will try to write an article on that case and on two others on whom I used the medicine. My faith in Ecthol is unlimited, and can only say the case above described, from a city of twenty-eight physicians, has increased my practice in that locality."—*Medical Brief.*

A. O. Stimpson, M. D., C. M., Thompson, Pa., says: "I have used and prescribed Celerina as a nervous sedative, in a sufficient number of cases to test its medical virtues, and by experience I find that it is by far the most effective anodyne compound that is made. It is especially adapted to such cases that wil not tolerate opiates, especially in neurasthenia and hysteric convulsions. I have also used it as a calmative in several cases of insomnia, brought on by over indulgence in the use of alcoholic stimulants. I have often combined it with Peacock's Bromides very effectually. Miss A. C., a young lady, inheriting an extremely nervous temperament from her mother, was treated by me 3 months ago for amenorrhea and chlorosis. Preparations of iron were prescribed for her with decided benefit, as a constitutional treatment, but she could get no rest at night, only when completely exhausted. Opiates of various kinds proved more of an excitant remedy than calmative. By the frequent and repeated use of bromides of potash, soda and ammonia, she would obtain rest when her stomach would tolerate the remedies, but Celerina proved to be the *sine qua non* in her case; the second dose scarcely ever failing to procure a protracted and refreshing sleep. Case 2. Mr. F. L., a professional house painter, occasionally afflicted with colica pictonum, immediately relieved of pain and trembling by repeated doses of Celerina given in milk. Case 3. Mrs. J. G., an aged lady, suffering from hemiplegia, attended with annoying formication in palsied limbs, was relieved of these disagreeable symptoms and of insomnia by the use of Celerina. Opiates of any kind failed to have any beneficial effect, and the bromides and preparations of valerian disagreed with her stomach. Case 4. Mr. S. S., an habitual toper, had had no sleep for three nights in sucession, where the stomach was in such a condition that it refused to tolerate alcoholic stimulants in any shape, was speedily relieved by the use of Celerina. Case 5. A. C., a young child, two years old, suffering from hydrocephalus, was greatly benefited by the use of Celerina as a nervine sedative, and is in a fair way to gain unlooked-for health.

Treatment of Chorea by Massive Doses of Arsenic.—Del Pozo (These de Paris; *Therap. Gazette,* August 15th) records thirty cases of chorea treated by massive doses of arsenic. He considers that these massive doses are far superior to treatment by antipyrin, as it is commonly employed, and states that there are two ways in which arsenic may be administered, namely, in small doses very gradually increased, and in large doses rapidly increased up to the point of intolerance, or, in other words, until the gastro-intestinal canal of the patient rebels, as manifested by vomiting and diarrhea. As soon as these symptoms are developed the dose is cut down day by day until one is obtained which the patient can bear. He asserts that such treatment usually produces cure within nine days, and that accident from this method is rarely met with. Four cases of arsenical neuritis are reported. Arsenical fever is rare; sometimes arsenical pigmentation occurs, but this speedily passes away as soon as the drug is stopped.—*B. M. J.*

The Pulse as a Sign of Neurasthenia.—Almost the only objective sign of neurasthenia is an irritable heart. Erben (*Wein. Klin. Woch.,* No. 24) has studied this condition especially, and has discovered the following peculiarity: If the patient is made to stoop, the pulse rate, instead of being quickened, as is normally the case after every movement of the body, suddenly slows down for three or four beats, and then gradually recovers or exceeds its original frequency. The stooping usually causes slight temporary cyanosis. This Erban attributes, not to rise of blood pressure, but to stimulation of the vagus by the increased venosity of the blood. Bending the head backward as far as possible also gives rise to the phenomenon, which is not elicited when the nervous system is healthy.

A True Nerve Tonic.—Dr. R. F. Williams, in the Charlotte *Medical Journal,* in considering this subject closes with following conclusions:

1. That for long continued use in conditions of weakened nerve power, is strychnine, arsenic, phosphorous and the hypophosphites are unsuitable on account of the ultimate depressant effect which their continued use may occasion, which should be avoided.

2. That in the glycero-phosphites we have preparations so nearly identical with the natural phosphorus compound of nerve substance as to be more readily appropriated by depressed nerve tissue than any other phosphorus preparations.

3. That this near identity of the glycero-phosphates with lecithin and the absence of nerve stimulation produced by their stimulation produced by their administration render them true nerve tonics.

4. That the success met with by those of the profession who have used these preparations entitles them to trial by the professional generally.

FOR SALE CHEAP.

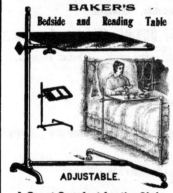
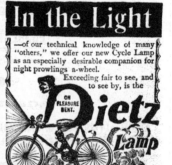
Please mention the Journal when you write to an advertiser.

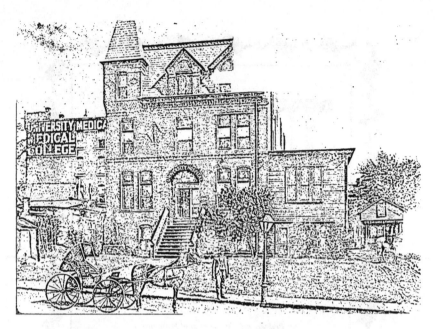

...UNIVERSITY HOSPITAL...

1005 Campbell Street, KANSAS CITY, MO.

The Trustees of the University Medical College take pleasure in announcing that they have renovated the hospital, carefully putting the building and its appointments in perfect sanitary condition. Have also added electric lights, electric cautery, electric galvanism, electric dry heat, X-ray apparatus for photography, etc. The hospital is not run in the exclusive interest of any school, church or individuals cut all physicians and friends are invited to send patients here, where individual rights and professional bourtesies will be observed.

######.....EXPENSES......

Board in private room, per week...$10 to $20
Two persons in one room, for each 7
Ward patients, each 6

######......EXTRAS .....

Use of operating-room for capital operations...$5
Minor operations.. 2
Dressings and Medicines at actual cost.

######......TRUSTEES......

For further information address.   **DR. FLAVEL B. TIFFANY, Manager,**
805 Mc Gee Street.

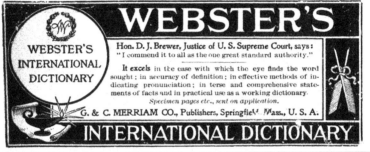
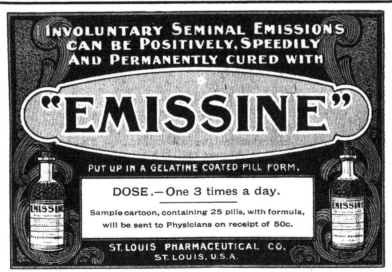
—27—

UNIVERSITY MEDICAL COLLEGE

OF KANSAS CITY, MO.

911 and 913 East Tenth Street.

College Opens September 11th, 1899, and Continues Six Months

FACULTY.

H. F. HEREFORD, M. D............ ....901 Forest Ave
    Emeritus Professor of Obstetrics.
JOHN K. SNELL, M. D. ....1124 Main St
    Emeritus Professor of Practice of Medicine.
R. R. HUNTER, M. D., Ph. D ....U. S. Army
    Emeritus Professor of Chemisty.
JAMES P. JACKSON. M. D ....1506 E. 8th St
    Emeritus Professor of Surgery.
J. M. ALLEN., A. B., M. D., L. L. D..........Liberty, Mo
    Professor of Principles and Practice of
    Medicine.
FLAVEL B. TIFFANY, M. D ....1235 Grand Av
    Professor of Ophthalmology and Otology.
GEORGE W. DAVIS, M. D..........Commerce Building
    Professor of Genito-Urinary and Venereal
    Diseases.
GEO HALLEY, M. D ....Ridge Building
    Professor of Principles and Practice of
    Surgery and Clinical Surgery.
JAMES E. LOGAN. M. D., President, 1208 Wyandotte
    Professor of Diseases of the Nose,
    Throat, and Chest.
ABEZ N. JACKSON, A. M., M. D ....Rialto Bldg
    Professor of Principles and Practice of
    Surgery and Clinical Surgery.
C. F. WAINRIGHT, M. D., Dean ....Altman Bldg
    Professor of Clinical Medicine and Physical
    Diagnosis.
S. G. GANT, M. D., Curator ....Rialto Bldg
    Professor of Rectal and Gastro-Intestinal Surgery.
JOHN PUNTON, M. D. Secretary ....Altman Bldg
    Professor of Nervous and Mental Diseases.
S. C. JAMES, M. D., Treasurer ....Times Bldg
    Professor of Principles and Practice of Medicine.
JOHN W. PERKINS, B. A., M. D..........Altman Bldg
    Professor of Principles and Practice of Surgery
    and Clinical Surgery.
JOHN WILSON. M. D ....504 Hall Bldg
    Professor of Hygiene and Preventive Medicine.
CLAY S. MERRIMAN, M. D................2811 Forest Av
    Professor of Diseases of Children.
A. M. WILSON, A. M. M. D ....908 Main St
    Professor of Physiology.
V W. GAYLE, M. D...............Deardorff Building
    Professor of Materia Medica and Therapeutics.
C. A. RITTER, M. D.......................... Altman Building
    Professor of Obstetrics.
CHAS. E. WILSON, M. D. ....Commerce Building
    Professor of Anatomy.
J. P. KASTER, M. D.........................Topeka, Kan
    Professor of Railway Surgery.
I. J. WOLF, M. D ....Rialto Bldg
    Professor of Bacteriology.
H. C. CROWELL, M. D.......... .... Altman Building
    Professor of Diseases of Women.
O. W. DULIN, M. D............................Rialto Building
    Professor of Pathology.

M. B. WARD, M. D........ ....Rialto Building
    Professor of Clinical Gynaecology at
    City Hospital.
A. H. CORDIER. M. D ....Rialto Bldg
    Professor of Abdominal Surgery.
J. P. KNOCHE, M. D... ....Ridge Building
    Professor of Dermatology.
BRUNO L. SULZBACHER, M. D. ......Commerce Bldg
    Professor of Histology.
W. M. CROSS, A. B...................... College Building
    Professor of Chemistry.
O. G. YOUNG, A. M., L. L. B. ....N. Y. Life Bldg
    Professor of Medical Jurisprudence.
S. GROVER BURNETT, M. D...............Rialto Bldg
    Professor of Physiology of the Nervous System
    and Clinical Neurology.
GEORGE W. GROVE, A. M., M. D.........Rialto Bldg
    Lecturer on Anatomy.
B. C. HYDE, A. B., M.D..............Altman Building
    Adjunct Professor and Chief Demonstrator
    of Anatomy.
H. D. JEROWITZ, M. D.............1233 Grand Avenue
    Lecturer on Materia Medica and Pharmacy.
MISS HAIDEE BERGER, M. D.......1223 Monroe Ave.
    Professor of Latin.
G. E. BELLOWS, A. M., M. D............Rialto Building
    Clinical Assistant to Chair of Ophthalmology.
CHET. McDONALD, M. D ....Rialto Building
    Assistant to Chair of Practice of Medicine.
J. N. SCOTT. M. D.........................Ridge Building
    Lecturer on Electro-Therapeutics.
L. W. LUSCHER, M. D............Ridge Building
    Assistant to Chair of Surgery.
W. J. FRICK, M. D.................... Commerce Bldg
    Assistant to Chair of Surgery.
S. H. WOODS, M. D ....Diamond Building
    Assistant to Chair of Practice of Medicine.
WALTER JACKSON, M. D........... Rialto Building
    Assistant to Chair of Clinical Medicine.
O. W. KRUEGER, M. D.............838 West Fifth Street
    Assistant to Chair of Bacteriology.
H. O. LEONARD, M. D.....................1214 Main Street.
    Assistant to Chair of Obstetrics.
S. S. LANDON. M. D ....Altman Bldg
    Assistant Chief Demonstrator of Anatomy.
*G. W. GROVE, A. M., M. D..............Rialto Building
*W. E. MONTGOMERY, M. D.................. Ridge Bldg
*E. W. SLUSHER, M. D ....908 Main Street
*F. L. SANDERS, M. D...................... 16th and Grand
*MARK MYERS, M. D...............12th and Grand Ave
*J. C. EGELSTON, M. D. .... Ridge Bldg
W. M. REED, M. D.....................1010 Main Street
    Clinical Assistant to Chair of Nose and Throat.
H. D. TUREMAN, M. D...................Altman Building
    Clinical Assistant to Chair of Diseases
    of Children.

*Demonstrators of Anatomy.

Graded Four Year Course. Every facility for Practical Study. Clinical advantages unsurpassed by any Western College. For catalogue or further particulars, apply to, C. F. WAINRIGHT, M. D., Dean, Altman Building, or JOHN PUNTON M. D., Secretary, Altman Building, Kansas City. Mo.

American Medical Association.

The annual meeting of the American Medical Association will be held in Atlantic City. N. J., June 5–8, 1900. It is confidently expected that the customary rates of one fare and one-third for the round trip will be made by all railroads for this occasion. For the convenience of our friends in Kansas City and territory west arrangements have been made to run a sleeping car through from Kansas City to Atlantic City, via Chicago & Alton R. R. to St. Louis, Big Four Route to Cincinnati, and Chesapeake & Ohio R. R. to Washington. The single trip rate from Kansas City to Atlantic City is $29.75. The charge for one double berth in through sleeping car as far as Philadelphia will be $8.00; two passengers may occupy one berth. A number of names have already been filed with the undersigned for space in this car and a most enjoyable trip is promised. The car will leave Kansas City at 9:15 p. m. Saturday evening, June 2nd, and berths may be reserved by writing to any one of the undersigned.

Any other information will be cheerfully furnished.

A. H. CORDIER, M. D.,
Rialto Building, Kansas City, Mo.
JNO. PUNTON, M. D.,
Altman Building, Kansas City, Mo.
or
ALEX. HILTON,
General Agent Passenger Dept. Chicago & Alton R. R.,
Kansas City, Mo.

Kansas City Medical College...

Established 1869.

Four Year Graded Course.

NEW BUILDING, NEW AND WELL EQUIPPED LABORATORIES,   **BEDSIDE INSTRUCTION IN MEDICINE SURGERY AND GYNECOLOGY.**

Annual Session Begins Sept. 12, and Continues Six Months.

——— FACULTY ———

S. S. Todd, M. D.,
David R. Porter, M. D.
Edw. W. Schauffler, A. M., M. D.,
Jefferson D. Griffith, M. D.,
John H. Van Eman, M. D.,
John H. Thompson, M. D.,
William C. Tyree, M. D.,
Joseph Sharp, M. D.,
Andrew L. Fulton, M. D.,
Charles H. Lester, M. D.
Henry O. Hanawalt, M. D.,
J. F. Binnie, A. M., M. D., C. M.
Robert T. Sloan, A. M., M. D.,
George C. Mosher, M. D.,
Franklin E. Murphy, M. D.

Thomas J. Beattie, M. D.,
Charles E. Clark, M. D.,
Hon. O. H. Dean, M. D.,
William Frick, M. D.,
J. J. Clausen, M. D.,
Edward H. Thrailkill, M. D.,
H. I. Hibbard, M. D.
Robert McE. Schauffler, M. D.,
Orrin H. Parker, M. D., Ph. G.,
Frank J. Hall, M. D.
A. Miller, M. D.
Frederick T. Van Eman, M. D.
Harry C. Hays, M. D.

For announcement and other information, address

Andrew L. Fulton, M. D., Dean.   **Franklin E. Murphy, M. D., Sec'y.**

New York Polyclinic Medical School and Hospital.

A CLYNICAL SCHOOL FOR GRADUATES IN MEDICINE AND SURGERY.

The New York Polyclinic is a school for teaching graduates the most recent methods of diagnosis and treatment in every department of medicine. The clinical material is abundant and the hospital wards adjoin the lecture rooms. Since the fire of 1896 a new building has been erected and thoroughly equipped and the Institution is now prepared to offer better facilities than ever. Students may enter at any time.

FACULTY.

SURGERY.—Robert H. M. Dawbarn, M. D., George R. Fowler M. D., John A. Wyeth, M. D., W. R. Townsend, M. D., James P. Tuttle, M. D., Charles H. Chetwood, M. D.

MEDICINE.—Isaac Adler, M. D., Wm. H. Katzenbach, M. D., W. W. VanValzah, M. D.

GYNECOLOGY.—J. Riddle Goffe, M. D., Morris Manges, M. D., Paul F. Munde, M. D., Wm. R. Pryor, M. D., W. Gill Wylie, M. D.

DISEASES OF CHILDREN.— L. Emmett Holt, M. D., August Seibert, M. D.

DERMATOLOGY.—Ed. B. Bronson, M. D., Andrew R. Robinson, M. D.

OPHTHALMOLOGY.—Wilbur B. Marple, M. D., David Webster, M. D., R. O. Born, M. D.

LARYNGOLOGY AND RHINOLOGY.—D. Bryson Delavah, M. D., Joseph W. Gleitsmann, M. D.

OTOLOGY.—Robert C. Myles, M. D., Oren D. Pomeroy, M. D., Fredrick Whiting, M. D.

DISEASES OF THE MIND AND NERVOUS SYSTEM.—Landon Carter Gray, M. D., B. Sachs, M. D.

OBSTETRICS.—Edward A. Ayres, M. D.

FOR FURTHER INFORMATION APPLY TO

W. R. TOWNSEND, Secretary.

214 TO 218 EAST 34th STREET.   *NEW YORK CITY*

Please mention the Journal when you write to an advertiser.

NEW YORK POST=GRADUATE MEDICAL SCHOOL AND HOSPITAL.

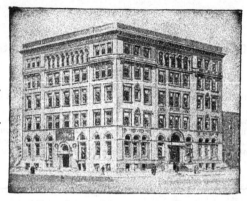

Eighteenth

Year.

Session of

1899-1900.

UNIVERSITY

OF THE

STATE OF

NEW YORK.

FACULTY

D. D. St. John Roosa. M. D., LL. D.
Andrew H. Smith, M. D.
William Oliver Moore, M. D.
Bache McE. Emmett, M. D.
Edward Kershner, M. D.
William H. Porter, M. D.
Stephen S. Burt, M. D.
Seneca D. Powell, M. D.
C. A. von Ramdohr, M. D.
Horace T. Hanks, M. D., LL. D.
Clarence C. Rice, M. D,
Graeme M. Hammond, M. D.
J. R. Nilsen, M. D.
George B. Fowler, M. D.
A. M. Phelps, M. D.
Henry D. Chapin, M. D.
O. B. Douglas, M. D.
J. B. Emerson, M. D.
Frederick Bagoe, Ph. B.
Farquhar Ferguson, M. D.
Reynold W. Wilcox, M. D., LL. D.
W. B. DeGarmo, M. D.
Daniel Lewis, M. D.
William J. Morton, M. D.
Hermann J. Boldt, M. D.
Augustus Caille, M. D.
Willy Meyer, M. D.
A. Palmer Dudley, M. D.
George M. Edebohls, M. D.
Francis Valk, M. D.
Ramou Guiteras, M. D.

Frank N. Lewis, M. D.
Leonard Weber, M. D.
Eugene Fuller, M. D.
Joseph Collins, M. D.
Edward S. Peck, M. D.
Samuel Lloyd, B. Sc., M. D.
James King Crook, M. D.
Ralph Waldo, M, D.
Robert Tuttle Morris, M. D.
Adolph Zeb, M. D.
Abbott Carson Combs, M. D.
John Dorning, M. D.
Frank Van Fleet, M. D.
Max Einhorn, M. D.
Achilles Edward Davis. M. D.
Theodore Dunham, M. D.
Warren Oscar Plimpton, M. D.
Wendell Christopher Phillips, M D.
Henry Turner Brooks, M. D.
James Brentano Clemens, M. D.
Abram Brothers, M. D.
Carter Standard Cole, M. D.
Franz Torek, M. D.
Henry B. Douglass, M. D.
John O. Polak, M. D.
Andrew von Grimm, M. D.
Charles O. Maisch, M. D.
W. Bedford Brown, M. D.
John McGrath, M. D.
Forbes Hawkes, M. D.

THE POST-GRADUATE MEDICAL SCHOOL AND HOSPITAL occupies the largest and best building for combined hospital and college purposes in the country. It is an eight-story fire-proof structure, containing accommodations for 175 patients. The Babies' Wards are an integral part of the institution, under its own roof, with beds for fifty-three patients. The new building has adequate accommodations for the personal instruction of large classes of practitioners, while the hospital facilities are equal to those of any hospital in the City of New York. Every opportunity, both in the Dispensary and Hospital is afforded in all departments of medicine and surgery. The major operations are performed in the amphitheater of the institution, which is fitted up in a manner to secure the best surgical results. Pathological and Histological Laboratories are also a part of the school. The Faculty are connected with many of the great hospitals and dispensaries in the city, where other clinics are held for the benefit of matriculates of the POST-GRADUATE MEDICAL SCHOOL. Practitioners may enter at any time.

Members of the profession who are visiting New York for a day or two will be heartily welcomed at the POST-GRADUATE SCHOOL, and if they desire to attend the clinics, a visitor's ticket, good for two days, will be furnished them on application to the Superintendent.

D. B. ST. JOHN ROOSA, M. D., LL. D., PRESIDENT.

SENECA D. POWELL, M. D., SECRETARY OF THE FACULTY.

ALEXANDER H. CANDLISH, SUPERINTENDENT.   Cor. Second Ave. and 20th St., New York City.

BENJAMIN B. LOWDEN, ASSISTANT SUPERINTENDENT,

Physicians coming to the School will please ask for the Supt. or Ass't. Supt.

Please mention the Journal when you write to an advertiser.

✳ Chicago Clinical School ✳

A Post-Graduate School of Medicine,

Surgery and all of the Specialties.

819 Harrison Street.

Advantages:

Located in the CENTER OF CHICAGO'S MEDICAL COLONY.
FULLY EQUIPPED FOR POST-GRADUATE INSTRUCTION in all branches of medicine and surgery.
LARGE HOSPITAL IN OUR OWN BUILDING accommodating 125 patients.
OPEN THE YEAR AROUND: ENTER AT ANY TIME with equal advantages.
Access to the numerous medical institutions located within a radius of 2 blocks of our building.
DAILY BULLETIN OF OPERATIONS to take place in all of the principal hospitals in this city.
Excellent courses in DISSECTION and SURGICAL ANATOMY ON CADAVER.
Opportunity to witness THREE POST-MORTEMS EACH WEEK.
EXCELLENT ADVANTAGES FOR LABRATORY WORK in all branches.
All surgical operations witnessed from CLOSE RANGE.
Every minute of your time from 9:00 a. m. to 6:00 p. m. fully and profitably occupied.
Access to the CLINICAL WORK done in COOK COUNTY HOSPITAL (1500 patients) located across the street from our building.
Opportunity afforded for witnessing EMERGENCY WORK during the day time and at night.
Students COME IN DIRECT CONTACT WITH PATIENTS making the examinations in all cases
UNLIMITED AMOUNT OF CLINICAL MATERIAL.
NUMBER OF MATRICULANTS LIMITED.

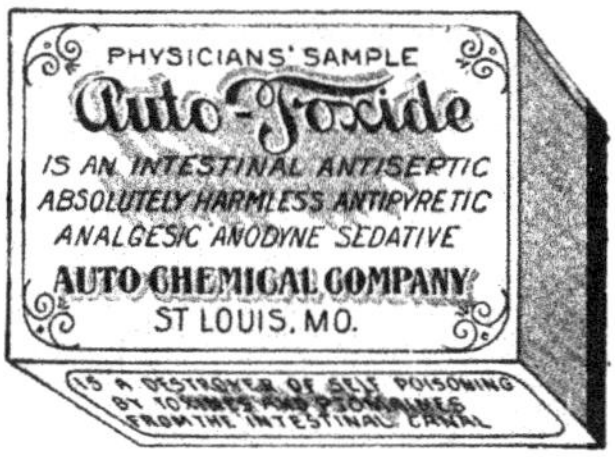

Courtesies of this Institution extended for two Days, to Visitors and prospective Matriculants.

Write for Illustrated Catalogue.   **W. L. NOBLE,** SECRETARY.

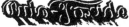
Please mention the Journal when you write to an advertiser.

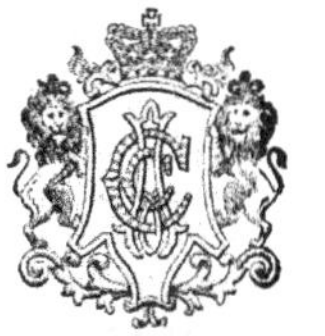

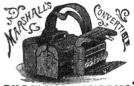
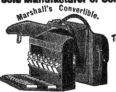
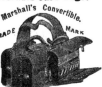
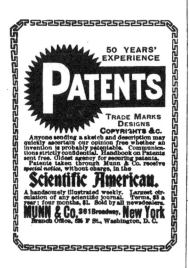
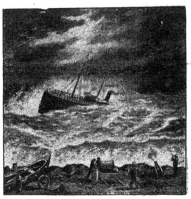
Please mention the Journal when you write to an advertiser.

HOT SPRINGS, ARKANSAS,

THE CARLSBAD OF AMERICA.
THE SARATOGA OF THE WEST.

VIA ———

DOUBLE DAILY TRAIN SERVICE.

MISSOURI PACIFIC RAILWAY.

Leaving ——— Kansas City at 9;50 and 10 a. m and 1:10 and 9:00 p. m.

Hot Springs, Arkansas has no equal in the United States for elegant hotels. The beautiful Park hotel; the Arlington, located on the United States government reservation, the hotel Eastman, the Monarch of the Glen, the Avenue hotel, Hotel Pullman, Waukesha, Great Northern and many other hotels and boarding houses of all grades, and suitahle for all sorts and conditions of men. There is no place of the kind in the country where everyone, no matter what his social, financial or physical condition may be, can find an abiding place perfectly adapted to his needs so readily as at Hot Springs.

Its baths, resorts and beautiful scenery in the heart of the Ozark mountains make it a delightful place of resort both winter, spring and summer. How to get to Hot Springs, Arkansas? See or address for full information in regard to excursion rates and train service, E. S. Jewett, Passenger and Ticket Agent, No. 901 Main St. (Sheidley Building,)' Kansas City, Mo. Remember the route! Via Missouri Pacific and St. Louis, Iron Mountain & Southern Railway.

H. C. TOWNSEND, G. P. A., Missouri Pacific Railway, St. Louis, Mo.

THE BEST LINE EAST

....VIA THE....

Burlington Route

Train leaves for
CHICAGO
6:10 p. m.
Daily.
Solid Vestibuled
Train,
Pullman Sleepers,
Chair Cars,
Dining Cars,
(a la carte,)
The finest service
out of Kansas City.

These
two
Trains
make connections
with all lines
for the
East and
South.

Train leaves for
ST. LOUIS
9:00 p. m.
Daily.
Solid Vestibuled
Train,
Pullman Sleeper
Compartment Sleeper,
and
Chair Cars
an
Elegant Train.

Ticket Office, 823 Main Street.

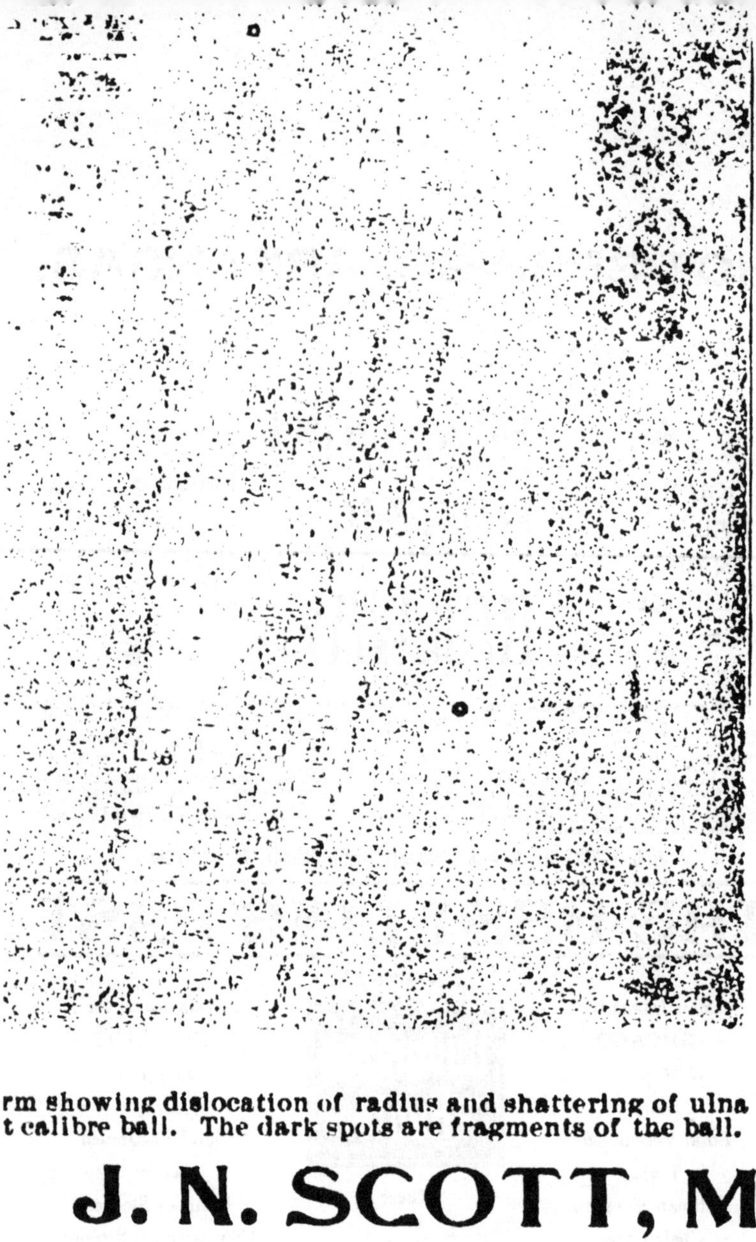

rm showing dislocation of radius and shattering of ulna by
t calibre ball. The dark spots are fragments of the ball.

J. N. SCOTT, M.

43

CONTENTS.

SYR. HYPOPHOS. CO., FELLOWS

Contains the Essential Elements—of the Animal Organization—Potash and lime:

The Oxidising Agents—Iron and Manganese;

The Tonics—Quinine and Strychnine;

And the Vitalizing Constituent—Phosphorus; the whole combined in the form of a Syrup with a **Slightly Alkaline Reaction.**

It Differs in its Effects from all Analogous Preparations and it possesses the important properties of being pleasant to the taste, easily borne by the stomach, and harmless under prolonged use.

It has Gained a Wide Reputation, particularly in the treatment of Pulmonary Tuberculosis, Chronic Bronchitis, and other affections of the respiratory organs. It has also been employed with much success in various nervous and debilitating diseases.

Its Curative Power is largely attributable to its stimulant, tonic, and nutritive properties, by means of which the energy of the system is recruited.

Its Action is Prompt; it stimulates the appetite and the digestion, it promotes assimilation, and it enters directly into the circulation with the food products.

The prescribed dose produces a feeling of buoyancy, and removes depression and melancholy ; *hence the preparation is of great value in the treatment of mental and nervous affections.* From the fact, also, that it exerts a double tonic influence, and induces a healthy flow of the secretions, its use is indicated in a wide range of diseases.

NOTICE--CAUTION.

The success of Fellows' Syrup of Hypophosphites has tempted certain persons to offer imitations of it for sale. Mr. Fellows, who has examined samples of several of these, **finds that no two of them are dentical,** and that all of them differ from the original in composition, in freedom from acid, reaction, in susceptibility to the effects of oxygen when exposed to light or heat, **in the property of retaining the strychnine in solution,** and in the medicinal effects.

As these cheap and inefficient substitutes are frequently dispensed instead of the genuine preparation, physicians are earnestly requested, when prescribing the Syrup, to write "Syr. Hypophos. **Fellows.**"

As a further precaution, it is advisable that the Syrup should be ordered in the original bottles; the distinguishing marks which the bottles (and the wrappers surrounding them) bear, can then be examined, and the genuineness—or otherwise—of the contents thereby proved.

Medical Letters may be addressed to

Mr. FELLOWS, 48 Vesey Street, New York.

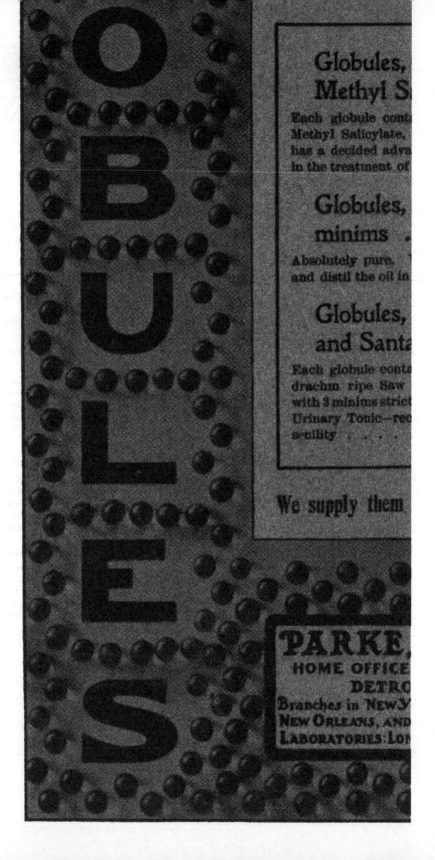

O B U L E S

WS - #0091 - 161123 - C0 - 229/152/5 - PB - 9780243062041 - Gloss Lamination